LONG-TERM CARE
FOR THE ELDERLY

Also of interest from the Urban Institute Press:

Medicare: A Policy Primer, by Marilyn Moon

Intergenerational Caregiving, edited by Alan Booth, Ann C. Crouter, Suzanne M. Bianchi, and Judith A. Seltzer

THE URBAN INSTITUTE PRESS
WASHINGTON, DC

LONG-TERM CARE FOR THE ELDERLY

ROBYN STONE

THE URBAN INSTITUTE PRESS
2100 M Street, N.W.
Washington, D.C. 20037

Library of Congress Cataloging-in-Publication Data

Stone, Robyn.
  Long-term care for the elderly / Robyn I. Stone.
      p. ; cm.
  Includes bibliographical references and index.
  ISBN 978-0-87766-770-4 (paper: alk. paper) 1. Older people—Long-term care—United States. 2. Older people—Medical care—United States. I. Urban Institute. II. Title.
  [DNLM: 1. Aged. 2. Long-term Care. 3. Health Services for the Aged. WT 31]
  RC954.3.S76 2011
  362.16—dc23

                                    2011013617

Printed in the United States of America
13 12 11   1 2 3 4 5

THE URBAN INSTITUTE is a non-profit, nonpartisan policy research and educational organization established in Washington, D.C., in 1968. Its staff investigates the social, economic, and governance problems confronting the nation and evaluates the public and private means to alleviate them. The Institute disseminates its research findings through publications, its web site, the media, seminars, and forums.

Through work that ranges from broad conceptual studies to administrative and technical assistance, Institute researchers contribute to the stock of knowledge available to guide decisionmaking in the public interest.

Conclusions or opinions expressed in Institute publications are those of the authors and do not necessarily reflect the views of officers or trustees of the Institute, advisory groups, or any organizations that provide financial support to the Institute.

Contents

Acknowledgments

I would first like to thank LeadingAge for providing me with the infrastructure and moral support to write this book over the past two years. Special thanks go to Natasha Bryant, Alisha Sanders, and Felita Kamara, who spent countless hours helping me to prepare the data tables and tracking down references. I also want to acknowledge the many professional colleagues who provided much of the literature that I synthesized in this volume. The community of long-term care researchers and policy analysts is strong and vibrant and continues to raise important policy issues as well as identify possible solutions. On a personal level, I must also thank my significant other, Robert, for sharing many weekends with me writing at the kitchen table. Finally, I want to express my gratitude to my grandmother for introducing me at an early age to the value of an aging society and for encouraging me to pursue my professional goals and aspirations in this field.

1

The Fundamentals of Long-Term Care

M rs. Smith, an 88-year-old widow with late-stage dementia, moved to a nursing home two years ago when the care she required became too complex for the assisted living facility in which she was residing. Mr. Jones, a 70-year-old retired janitor with diabetes and hypertension, lives in an inner-city, publicly subsidized senior high-rise building, takes 10 medications for his chronic diseases, and receives Medicaid-funded personal care in his apartment twice a week. Although his elderly neighbor also needs this type of assistance and cannot afford to pay out of pocket for these services, her low income is, unfortunately, just above the financial threshold that would qualify her for Medicaid coverage. Ms. Perez, a married, 50-year-old manager of a small business in a Midwest rural town, lives with her husband, a teenage daughter, and her 83-year-old mother-in-law who moved in with the family after being discharged from a skilled nursing facility following rehabilitation treatment for a stroke.

The common thread connecting these scenarios is that all of these individuals have been faced with the need for long-term care and the complex decisions associated with getting services. Today, an estimated 6 million people age 65 and older—almost one in six older adults—need long-term care (Kaye, Harrington, and LaPlante 2010). Over 182 billion public and private dollars are spent on services and supports to help minimize, rehabilitate, or compensate for the loss of chronically disabled elderly individuals' physical or cognitive functioning (The Lewin Group 2010). Family members—primarily spouses and adult daughters—and friends provide the majority of services and supports. Those using the formal care system typically find themselves navigating a confusing, fragmented array of funding sources, policies, and programs that do not facilitate easy service access and use.

This book is a primer that provides an overview of long-term care, including what it is, why it is an important policy concern, and the key issues that policymakers, providers, consumers, and other stakeholders are struggling with today and will confront in the future. While the majority of the long-term care population is age 65 or older, 45 percent are under age 65, including individuals with physical, intellectual, and developmental disabilities and children with special care needs (Kaye et al. 2010). These groups form an important subset of the long-term care population, particularly among those living in community-based, noninstitutional settings. The issues and trends related to this diverse population, however, are beyond the scope of this book. Although many of the long-term care needs are similar across both age groups, the goals and preferences of younger people with disabilities are often different from their elderly counterparts (e.g., participating in or returning to school or work). Elderly individuals are also more likely than those under age 65 to need long-term care services that interface with the acute and subacute care system. In addition, the risk of needing long-term care is much greater for those age 65 and older. For these reasons, this primer focuses on long-term care for the elderly population.

Defining Long-Term Care

Long-term care encompasses a broad range of services and supports intended primarily to help chronically disabled elderly individuals to function as independently as possible for as long as possible. The need for long-term care emerges from chronic and debilitating medical conditions that can occur at birth, during developmental stages, or from accidents. Services provide assistance with basic activities of daily living (ADLs)—dressing, bathing, toileting, eating, and getting in and out of bed or chairs—as well as help with instrumental activities of daily living (IADLs), including household chores like meal preparation and cleaning; life management tasks, such as shopping, money management and medication management; and transportation. They include both hands-on, direct care and standby or supervisory human assistance. Long-term care also encompasses the use of assistive devices (e.g., canes, walkers, wheelchairs) and technology, such as computerized medication reminders and electronic monitoring systems that help individuals with dementia avoid falling or wandering. Building ramps, adding grab bars, and making other modifications to the home are also often included within the definition of long-term care.

An increasing proportion of individuals needing long-term care, particularly those in nursing homes, are medically complex, requiring attention to their medical and their functional needs arising from multiple chronic conditions, such as heart disease, chronic obstructive pulmonary disease (COPD), and diabetes, as well as management of problem behaviors resulting from dementia and other cognitive impairments. Long-term care also includes intense short-term medical, rehabilitative, and therapeutic care to patients following a hospitalization—typically referred to as "post-acute care." These services can be provided in a nursing facility, inpatient hospital rehab unit, long-term care hospital, or an individual's home (Alliance for Quality Nursing Home Care 2009). The primary goal of post-acute care is restorative and most of these individuals receive services for a short time.

Factors Affecting the Increased Focus on Long-Term Care Policy

Four factors are driving the increased attention on long-term care policy. The first is the aging of the population and how that demographic trend will influence the demand for services. The second is the concern about the costs of long-term care to individuals, families, and society and the impact of current and future demand on Medicaid, Medicare, and other public programs that cover a large portion of the costs of long-term care in the United States. The third is the short- and long-term availability of family caregivers and a well-trained, stable formal workforce to provide the services and to meet the increased demand projected over the next 30 years. The fourth is a continuing concern about the quality of care delivered in nursing homes and, with the expansion of publicly subsidized home and community-based care, an increasing focus on quality issues in these settings.

The Demographic Imperative: Aging and Disability

The aging of the society is the major factor behind the increased interest in and concern for long-term care policy since the risk of becoming disabled and needing long-term care increases substantially with age. Analyses of data from the 2005 Survey of Income and Program Participation and the 2004 National Nursing Home Survey indicate that only 0.9 percent of children less than 18 years old and 2.3 percent of Americans age 18 to 64 had long-term care needs as measured by the presence of ADL and/or IADL limitations (Kaye et al. 2010). In contrast, 13.4 percent of the population age 65 years and older needed long-term care.

Among the elderly population, the need for long-term care also increases substantially with age. Defining the need for long-term care as the inability to perform one or more of five physical activities (stooping or kneeling, reaching over one's head, writing or grasping small objects, walking two to three blocks, and lifting 10 pounds), researchers found that in 2007, both men and women were more likely to need assistance as they aged (Interagency Forum on Aging Related Statistics 2010). A little over one in five women and 13 percent of men age 65 to 74 were functionally disabled; the comparable estimates for those age 75

Figure 1.1. Percent of U.S. Population Needing Long-Term Care, by Age, 2004–2005

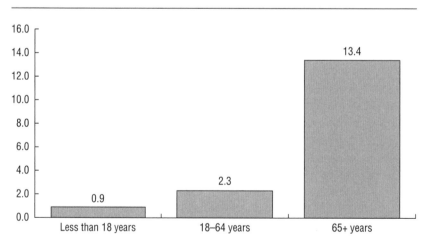

Source: Kaye et al. (2010); 2005 Survey of Income and Program Participation and the 2004 National Nursing Home Survey.

to 84 were 35.1 and 23.1 percent. Among women and men age 85 and older, the proportion increases substantially to 55.9 and 40.4 percent, respectively. Elderly black Medicare enrollees are more likely than the other racial groups to be disabled; elderly black women are the most likely to be disabled.

Today, the United States is a relatively young country with 13 percent of its population age 65 and older, on par with Australia, New Zealand, Montenegro, and Uruguay (Population Reference Bureau 2009). In contrast, 23 percent of Japanese and one out of five Italians and Greeks are age 65 and older. By 2030, however, 19 percent of the population in the United States will be elderly, as all of the baby boomers will have moved into the elderly population (Vincent and Velcoff 2010). Between 2007 and 2030, the population age 65 and older is projected to grow by 89 percent, more than four times as fast as the population as a whole (Houser, Fox-Grage, and Gibson 2009). Most of this growth will be among the young old (age 65 to 74) because baby boomers (those born between 1946 and 1964) will start turning 65 in 2011. From 2030 on, the proportion of people age 65 and older will be relatively stable, though the absolute number is projected to continue to grow.

Growth in the 85 and older population—the group most likely to need long-term care—will significantly affect the demand for long-term care. This "oldest old" population is expected to increase by 74 percent between 2007 and 2030 (Houser et al. 2009). The number of people in this age category is projected to grow from 5.8 million in 2010 to 8.7 million in 2030 and, by 2050—when the baby boomers have all entered the "oldest old" group—the number is projected to reach 19 million (Vincent and Velcoff 2010).

Since many long-term care policy decisions are made at the state level, these demographic trends vary by state. Florida, the oldest state with 17.4 percent of its population age 65 and older in 2008, will remain in that status at 27.1 percent elderly in 2030. Alaska, on the other hand, at 7.3 percent age 65 and older in 2008, will remain the youngest state in 2030 with 14.7 percent of its population classified as elderly (Interagency Forum on Aging-Related Statistics 2010; Houser et al. 2009). The states with the largest proportion of "oldest old" are likely to experience the greatest stress on public resources, such as the Medicaid program (the primary public payer for long-term care described in detail in chapter 4). In 2007, Florida, Iowa, North Dakota, and South Dakota had the largest proportion of oldest old, with over 2.5 percent of their populations

Figure 1.2. Percentage of Medicare Enrollees Age 65+ Unable to Perform One or More Physical Functions, by Age and Race, 2007

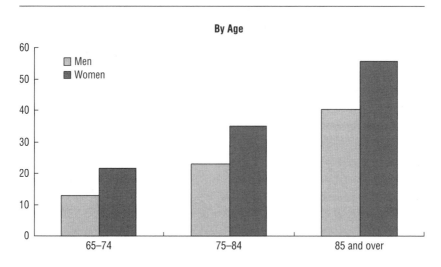

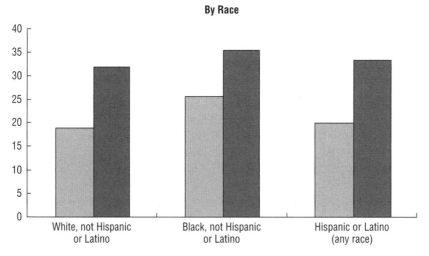

Source: Centers for Medicare and Medicaid Services, Medicare Current Beneficiary Survey.

Notes: The five physical functions include stooping or kneeling, reaching over one's head, writing or grasping small objects, walking two to three blocks, and lifting 10 pounds. Reference population data refer to Medicare enrollees.

age 85 and over. By 2030, 36 states and the District of Columbia will have at least 2.5 percent of their populations in the "oldest old" category (Houser et al. 2009).

Rural states with high concentrations of elderly people face particularly serious service-access challenges due to a dearth of younger people (who have moved to more urban locations) available to provide the services and a lack of proximity of the elderly population to services that do exist. In 2007, one in five people age 65 and older lived in rural, nonmetropolitan areas where services—and home and community-based options in particular—are typically harder to find (Houser et al. 2009).

Can Society Afford Long-Term Care?

The need for long-term care (LTC) is a relatively rare event. It is estimated that a little less than one in three Americans turning age 65 in 2005 will not need care during their remaining lifetimes (Kemper, Komisar, and Alexcih 2005). For individuals who need long-term care, however, the cost of services is often financially out of reach. In 2010, the median annual cost of nursing home care was $67,525 for a semi-private room and $75,190 for a private room (Genworth Financial 2010). The national median annual cost for assisted living was $38,220; the comparable estimate for adult day services was $15,600. Home care nurses hired through an agency charge between $20 and $40 an hour; the services of an agency-employed personal care attendant or home care aide average between $12 and $18 an hour and half that amount for services purchased in the "underground" market. Kemper and colleagues (2005) have estimated that 30 percent of those turning 65 in 2005 will spend at least $25,000 on long-term care over their remaining years; 16 percent will spend $100,000 or more.

As will be described in more detail in chapter 4, most individuals have not saved enough during their working years to cover these costs, and only a minority have purchased long-term care insurance. Most individuals rely primarily or solely on their family members and other unpaid helpers, such as friends and neighbors, for assistance. Low-income elderly individuals or those who have spent down their income and assets to a particular level are entitled to nursing home coverage and, depending on the state, may receive home care services through Medicaid—the joint federal/state health insurance program for the poor. Individuals with rehabilitation needs following a hospitalization may receive coverage for these services on a short-term basis through Medicare—the universal

Figure 1.3. Distribution of LTC Spending for Individuals Turning Age 65 in 2005

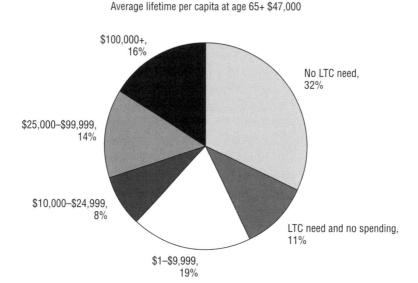

Average lifetime per capita at age 65+ $47,000

$100,000+, 16%

No LTC need, 32%

$25,000–$99,999, 14%

$10,000–$24,999, 8%

LTC need and no spending, 11%

$1–$9,999, 19%

Source: Kemper et al. (2005).
LTC = long-term care

health insurance program for the elderly and younger disabled. In 2007, of the total $190.4 billion in estimated spending for nursing home and home health care for the elderly and younger people with disabilities, Medicaid and other public funds paid for 42 percent and Medicare paid for 25 percent (Hartman et al. 2009). Given the portion of the long-term care bill paid for with public dollars, it is not surprising that policymakers at the federal and state levels are concerned about the short- and long-term financial viability of the Medicaid and Medicare programs (National Governors Association 2010). To deal with budget short-falls following the 2008 recession, at least 25 states and the District of Columbia cut home care services to the elderly and younger disabled in 2010 (McNichol, Oliff and Johnson 2010). Many states have also proposed nursing facility rate reductions, exacerbating chronic under-funding of these organizations (Alliance for Quality Nursing Home Care 2010). Escalating Medicare costs, including the costs of post-acute skilled nursing care and home health care, are also raising concerns about this segment of long-term care among federal policy officials. The total number of Medicare post-acute beneficiaries grew by 21 percent between 1999 and 2007; their expenditures increased by 75 percent (Ng, Harrington, and Kitchener 2010). Policymakers, providers, and consumers acknowledge that the projected increase in demand for long-term care over the next 20 years poses a significant challenge to the long-term sustainability of Medicaid, Medicare, and other state and local programs that subsidize long-term care.

Who Will Care?

The other major issue driving long-term care policy discussions is the question of who is and will be available to deliver care to meet current and future demand. Given the pivotal role that families play in providing care, the continued availability of family caregivers is critically important to public policymakers who are concerned about the future solvency of Medicaid and other public programs. There are uncertainties, however, about the extent to which family members will be willing and available to continue to be the primary long-term care provider. Trends such as rising divorce rates, increased rates of childlessness, declining family sizes, and rising employment rates of married women suggest that family caregiver availability is likely to decline in the future (Gonyea 2009). One gross measure of the availability of informal caregivers is the ratio of the population in the average caregiving range—age 50 to 64—to the population age 85 and older. In 1990, that ratio was 11 to 1; by 2050, there is projected to be only four potential caregivers for every elderly person in the "old old" category (Vincent and Velkoff 2010).

These combined trends indicate that the demand for long-term care services, particularly formal care, will grow over the next several decades. Many policymakers, providers, direct-care worker associations, and consumer groups agree that the formal long-term care workforce is already in crisis (Stone and Harahan 2010). As will be described in more detail in chapter 5, the crisis is reflected in labor shortages; rapid staff turnover among administrators, clinicians, and direct care workers; the inability of many consumers to find willing providers outside their families; and grave concerns about the quality of the workforce and how that translates into quality of care (Institute of Medicine [IOM] 2008; Harahan and Stone 2009). Without significant policy interventions that help to expand the supply of administrative, clinical, and direct-care workers;

invest in workforce education and training initiatives; and make long-term care jobs more competitive, the situation is likely to worsen over the next 30 years.

Ensuring Quality in Long-Term Care

Another issue that has drawn attention to long-term care policy is concern about the quality of the services being delivered. Research findings, media reports, and other anecdotal evidence have highlighted quality problems in nursing homes for over two decades (IOM 1986, 2001; Wiener, Freiman, and Brown 2007) and despite improvement in such areas as restraint reduction, substantial concerns remain (Castle and Ferguson 2010; Werner and Konetzka 2010). As states expand their home and community-based care programs and attempt to relocate segments of the nursing home population to community-based alternatives, concerns about the quality of long-term care in noninstitutional settings have surfaced. As chapter 7 will review in detail, a variety of public- and private-sector strategies and specific initiatives have been used and continue to be explored to help ensure that quality services are being delivered.

The Primer

In the following chapters, this primer describes the fundamentals of long-term care provided to the elderly population in the United States. The book begins with an overview of the current long-term care system, including the types of services provided under the rubric of long-term care and the settings in which the care is provided. Chapter 3 describes the elderly long-term care population, including the overall demand for services and supports, key characteristics of those who need and use the services, and measures of unmet need. The following three chapters address the "triple knot" of long-term care policy—who pays for long-term care, who provides long-term care, and how services are delivered (Stone 2006a). Chapter 7 summarizes strategies the public and private sectors use to ensure quality services are delivered across all long-term care settings. Finally, the primer concludes with speculation about what long-term care policy and the system might look like in 2030, when the age wave reaches its peak.

2

The Long-Term Care System for the Elderly

T he long-term care system for the elderly population, with a few exceptions (see chapter 6 for examples), is really not a system. Rather, it is an array of personal care, health care, and social services and supports provided in various settings over a sustained period to persons with chronic conditions and functional limitations (IOM 2001; Stone 2006a). As noted in chapter 1, this primer focuses on the largest subset of that population—individuals age 65 and older who have long-term care needs.

Defining Long-Term Care

The major goal of long-term care is to minimize, rehabilitate, or compensate for the loss of independent physical or mental functioning and to maximize the quality of life for chronically disabled elderly people. Functional limitations are typically assessed as limitations in activities of daily living that reflect an individual's capacity for self-care and personal hygiene. They usually refer to five basic functions: dressing, bathing, eating, using the toilet, and transferring in and out of bed or chairs. Functional limitations are also assessed in terms of need for help with instrumental activities of daily living, which entail more complex tasks that enable an individual to live independently in the community.

These include the ability to perform household chores like meal preparation, cleaning, and doing the laundry; the ability get around independently outside one's own home; and the ability to perform important life management tasks, such as shopping, financial management, medication management, and using the telephone.

Personal Care

Personal care is primarily low-tech in nature and includes assistance with ADLs and IADLs that is not required to be provided by a licensed professional. Services include both hands-on and stand-by or supervisory human assistance. Personal care may also include supports such as canes and walkers and technology such as computerized medication reminders. Home modifications like building ramps, grab bars, and easy-to-use door handles are also frequently included in the definition of personal care services.

Health Care

Health care includes medical, nursing, and other services provided by physicians, nurses, medical social workers, therapists, and nursing aides (under nurse supervision) who address the skilled-care needs of the elderly long-term care population. Much of this skilled care is provided to individuals in nursing facilities, a long-term care hospital or inpatient rehabilitation facility or the person's own home after an acute hospital admission (Alliance for Quality Nursing Home Care 2009). This care—referred to as "post-acute"—is delivered for a relatively short time (see the section on Medicare in chapter 4 for a fuller discussion). In 2009, Medicare spent $45 billion on home health care and skilled nursing facility services, representing 9 percent of all Medicare expenditures and 18 percent of all long-term care expenditures (Kaiser Family Foundation [KFF] 2010).

Long-stay nursing home residents with medically complex needs and their counterparts living in home and community-based settings also need medical or skilled nursing services to address their chronic health care needs in addition to their functional needs. Many elderly people spend their final days in a nursing home; almost 7 in 10 people with dementia die in that setting (Mitchell et al. 2005). An increasing number of terminally ill nursing home residents and individuals living in home and community-based settings are choosing to use the Medicare hospice benefit that includes a range of palliative care services, such as pain and symptom management, in lieu of more aggressive interventions (Huskamp et al. 2010; Meier, Lim, and Carlson 2010).

Social Services

Social services are diverse and include linking people to a range of community resources and services, assisting in resolving family or financial problems associated with the need for long-term care, providing congregate or home-delivered meals, and arranging social and educational activities (IOM 2001). Transportation is also an important service within the rubric of social services.

The Medical Care/Long-Term Care Interface

People who need long-term care are also more likely than their non-disabled peers to need medical care to address problems related to both acute and chronic conditions. This is illustrated by the dramatic difference in Medicare expenditures for the two populations. The average annual Medicare expenditures for elderly people with no long-term care needs in 2005 were $4,289. The comparable expenditures for those with one or more ADL limitations and those with three or more ADL limitations were $14,775 and $18,902, respectively (Avalere Health 2008).

Unfortunately, for the long-term care population with significant medical care needs, neither practice patterns nor payment systems provide well for special needs and situations (see chapter 4 for a more detailed discussion). Medicare—the primary payer for medically related services for the elderly population—and Medicaid—the primary payer for long-term care services—are not integrated (with the few exceptions, described in chapter 6). The payment streams have created silos of care that are not person-centered and that are not organized to meet their service needs in a holistic manner. This lack of integration makes navigating the system difficult for both individuals and their family members.

Where Is Long-Term Care Provided?

Long-term care is provided in a range of settings, depending on the recipient's needs and preferences, the availability of informal support, and the

Figure 2.1. Medicare Parts A and B per Capita Spending, 2005

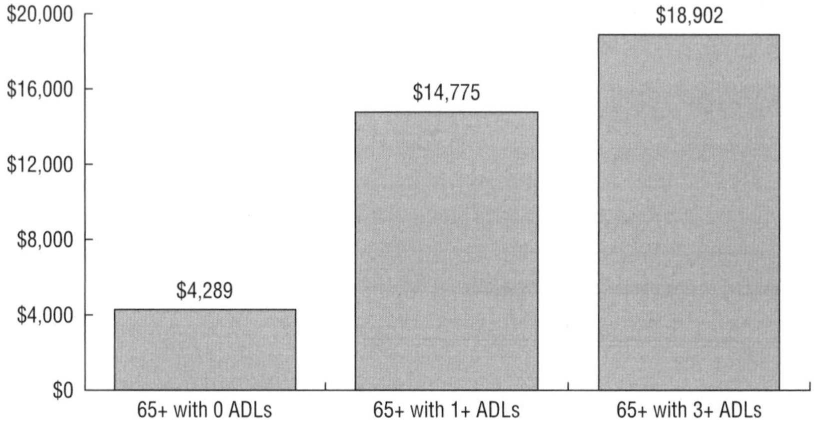

Source: Avalere Health (2008).
ADL = activity of daily living

source of reimbursement. Much gerontological literature refers to a continuum of care, identifying the nursing home as the most restrictive and one's own home as the least restrictive setting. The literature also stresses the appropriateness of a setting, assuming that strategies exist for matching the individual and the setting.

Some researchers have challenged the "continuum" and "appropriateness" paradigms (see, for example, Kane, Kane, and Ladd 1998; Stone 2006a), arguing that services can be delivered appropriately in any setting, depending on a constellation of individual, familial, and policy factors. One's own home, for example, can be as restrictive as a nursing home, if an individual is homebound and isolated and is not getting the services that would facilitate independence. Furthermore, appropriateness is subjective and should not be invoked to prevent individuals from making their own choices, which are often paramount to them.

Nursing Home

The nursing home—or nursing facility, as Medicaid and Medicare refer to this setting—is the institutional setting for elderly individuals who need long-term care.

In 2010, 15,683 nursing homes were certified by Medicare or Medicaid, down from 16,765 a decade ago (American Health Care Association [AHCA] 2010). Although the exact number of all private-pay nursing homes is unknown, it is believed to be a small fraction of all nursing facilities. There were approximately 1.7 million certified beds in 2010 with the median occupancy rate for certified beds at 87.4 percent.

In 2008, proprietary homes accounted for 67 percent of all facilities; 27 percent were nonprofit and the remainder were government sponsored (CMS 2009). All three ownership categories experienced declines in numbers between 2004 and 2008, but the rates of decrease among nonprofit and government facilities were much greater than among for-profit facilities (9, 8, and 1 percent, respectively).

Nursing homes care for both long-stay and short-stay populations. The long-stay elderly population is physically and, increasingly, cognitively impaired; a large proportion of the long stayers also have medically complex conditions and are likely to be taking multiple medications (see chapter 3 for a description of nursing home populations). Long-term care in a nursing facility can be very costly for these long-stay individuals. In 2008, the average annual private-pay cost of care in a nursing home was about $77,400 and as high as $125,000 in the most expensive markets (MetLife Mature Market Institute 2008). As chapter 4 will describe in more detail, the individual, his or her family, or the Medicaid program is likely to pay the costs of the nursing home stay out of pocket (Alexcih 2006).

Nursing homes are also the dominant provider of Medicare post-acute care services, treating more than half (52 percent) of all Medicare hospital discharges that require post-acute care (Alliance for Quality Nursing Home Care 2009). Home health agencies care for a little less than 37 percent of the discharges and only 12 percent are cared for in either inpatient rehabilitation facilities or long-term care hospitals.

Home and Community-Based Care

"Home and community-based care" is a catch-all phrase that refers to a wide range of noninstitutional long-term care settings, including the private homes/apartments of care recipients or their families and various types of residential care alternatives.

Home Care. The majority of elderly people who need long-term care live at home, either in their own homes or apartments, with or without

Figure 2.2. Share of Medicare Hospital Post-Acute Discharges by Provider, 2006

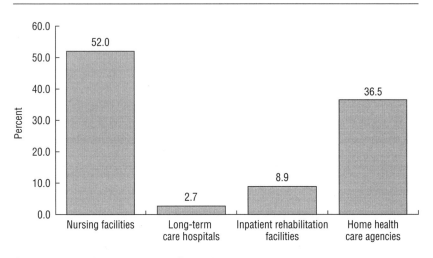

Source: Alliance for Quality Nursing Home Care (2009).

a spouse, or in the home of a close relative, such as a daughter. In this setting, a range of paid and unpaid services may be provided, including home health care and personal care.

Most individuals prefer to remain at home for as long as possible. Forty-one percent of individuals responding to a 2007 poll on long-term care believed that people deteriorate after nursing home placement. Only 4 percent said they would prefer a nursing home if they needed long-term care, 17 percent would choose assisted living, 53 percent would prefer care at home, and 21 percent would move in with family (KFF 2007). Furthermore, given the high costs of nursing home care and assisted living (see chapter 1), the home is the most affordable setting for many older adults and their families. The affordability is due, in large part, to the fact that adult daughters, spouses, and other family members and friends provide most of the care on an unpaid basis (see chapter 4).

Long-term care provided in the home runs the gamut from medically oriented skilled nursing care and rehabilitation to personal care and other supportive services. Home health care includes skilled nursing, physical and occupational therapy, and assistance (under nurse supervision) with personal care (i.e., ADL and IADL help). In 2009, there were 10,581 Medicare-certified home health agencies (National Association of Home

Care & Hospice 2010). Just over 8 percent of Medicare beneficiaries received some Medicare home health care visits in 2006, with an average of 35 visits per beneficiary. The state variation in the percentage of Medicare beneficiaries receiving home health care ranged from a low of 1.9 percent in Hawaii to a high of 11.4 percent in Louisiana (Houser, Fox-Grage, and Gibson 2009).

As noted in the introductory section of this chapter, a range of personal care and social services is provided in individual homes that includes assistance with ADLs and IADLs, home-delivered meals, care management to link individuals with community-based services, and special transportation. Often, people need home modifications and adaptations to remain independent in their own homes and communities (Pynoos, Feldman, and Ahrens 2004). Adaptations to individual homes include the installation of kitchen and bathroom cabinets that can accommodate wheelchair-bound individuals, wide bathroom and shower entries, shower and tub grab bars, door handles that are user-friendly for people with arthritis, and ramps.

Residential Care Alternatives. This category encompasses places and care arrangements that provide housing and services to older adults (and younger people) with varying degrees of disability and long-term care need. The terms that are often used include assisted living, board and care, and adult foster homes. Community-based residential care tends to be regarded as an option for individuals who may not need a nursing-home level of assistance but who can no longer remain in their own homes. It is often seen as a substitute for living at home and as the next step in a downward trajectory toward nursing home placement. The hallmark services tend to be assistance with IADLs, such as meals and housekeeping, and some personal care. Beyond these services, there is no consensus about what constitutes "residential care" among policymakers, providers, and researchers.

In contrast to nursing homes, which the federal government licenses and regulates because they receive significant Medicare and Medicaid reimbursement, state and local jurisdictions handle residential care. Since there is no consensus on the definition of residential care, the nomenclature as well as the nature and scope of services vary tremendously. Although many states use the term assisted living to cover almost every type of group residential care on the continuum between nursing homes and individual homes, for many stakeholders, the term *assisted living* represents a unique model of residential care that differs from traditional

Table 2.1. Adult Foster Care and Similar Residential Settings

Settings	Characteristics
Adult foster care homes, adult residential care homes, small group homes	• Private home in a residentially zoned neighborhood • No more than five or six older persons with physical disabilities per facility • No more than two residents to a room • Nonmedical services, such as meals, medication supervision or reminders, or help with ADLs • May provide some skilled nursing services, but not 24-hour skilled nursing care
Board and care facilities, large group homes	• Dormitory-style or ward-type facility • Four or more beds per facility • Three to four people may share a room • Mixed population • Nonmedical services, such as meals, medication supervision or reminders, or help with ADLs • May provide some skilled nursing services, but not 24-hour skilled nursing care
Assisted living facilities with private or semiprivate rooms	• Facility with private or semiprivate rooms • Each facility has four or more residents • Lockable room doors are permitted • Mainly serve only frail older adults • Freestanding facility • Basic level of care: provides meals, medication supervision, personal care, leisure activities, housekeeping, and laundry services • High level of care: provides RN/LPNs on staff. Extensive admission and retention criteria and high resident acuity

Source: Mollica, Sims-Kastelein, Cheek, et al. (2009).
ADL = activity of daily living, RN = registered nurse, LPN = licensed practical nurse

types of residential settings, such as board and care (Mollica, Sims-Kastelein, and O'Keefe 2007). In 2007, states reported 38,373 licensed residential care facilities with 974,585 units or beds.

Board and Care Homes. This residential care alternative tends to be a small, nonmedical community-based facility that typically provides at least two meals a day and routine protective oversight to one or more unrelated individuals with some level of functional disability. According to the last comprehensive study of this setting conducted in the mid-1990s, board and care homes are licensed and regulated under more than 25 different names; many more are unlicensed (Hawes, Wildfire, and Lux 1993). The physical character of the typical board and care home is institutional, with two to four people sharing a bedroom and as many as 8 to 10 residents sharing a bathroom (Mollica et al. 2007).

Assisted Living. Although no there is no single agreed-upon definition of assisted living, the term is used to connote a "residential setting that provides 24 hour supervision, provision and oversight of personal and supportive services, health-related services, social services, recreational activities, meals, housekeeping, laundry, and transportation" (Han, Sirrocco, and Remsburg 2003). In Oregon and later in other states, policymakers who were concerned about the institutional character of board and care homes developed a new licensing category called assisted living. In contrast to board and care, the philosophy of this category emphasized privacy (e.g., access to one's own room and bathroom) and the ability to have greater control over daily activities (Kane et al. 1998; Stone and Reinhard 2007).

A recent study of the assisted living market estimated that in 2007 there were 11,276 assisted living facilities with 839,746 units nationwide (Stevenson and Grabowksi 2010). The study researchers limited their supply data to facilities with 25 or more units, in an attempt to focus on facilities purposely built to be assisted living and to exclude adult foster care and small board and care homes. As of 2007, 29 states and the District of Columbia reported they include provisions regarding assisted living concepts, such as privacy, autonomy, and decisionmaking, in their residential care standards (Mollica et al. 2007). Fifteen states and the District of Columbia have regulations that address the need for an approach or process for negotiating disagreements about residents' autonomy and risk taking and providers' concerns about risk. Most states view assisted living facilities as licensed settings in which services are delivered. Four states (Connecticut, Maine, Minnesota, and New Jersey), however, define assisted living as a service—rather than a place—that may be provided in various settings, which do not have to be licensed.

As Mollica and colleagues (2007) note, one of the attractive philosophical tenets of assisted living is that it allows "aging in place"; as an individual ages and becomes more disabled, additional services can be provided so that the person does not have to move to a nursing home. State regulations specify allowable services and the minimum services that must be provided, including whether these facilities can provide skilled nursing care. These regulations, however, do not require the facilities to provide the full range of allowable services. There is, in fact, wide variation in how much skilled nursing and other health-related services are provided that would assist very disabled elderly residents to remain in the facility rather than moving to a "higher level of care" setting (Hawes et al. 2003).

Growth in assisted living has been driven in large part by consumer preference. While only 4 percent of respondents to a 2007 public opinion poll indicated that they would choose a nursing home if they needed long-term care, 17 percent reported that they would chose assisted living (KFF 2007). And at an average annual cost of $34,000, assisted living may seem like a bargain compared with the average $74,000 per year for a semiprivate room in a nursing home (Genworth Financial 2010). In contrast to the nursing home sector, where facilities are heavily dependent on public dollars, the assisted living sector has relied primarily on private resources and is an option mainly for middle- and upper-income individuals. Stevenson and Grabowski's market analysis (2010) supports this trend, finding that assisted living facilities are disproportionately located in areas with higher educational attainment, income, and housing wealth.

To date, states have been cautious about expanding Medicaid coverage for services provided in assisted living, and one recent estimate is that only 115,000 Medicaid recipients received services in this setting in 2007 (Mollica et al. 2007). Only a few states, such as Oregon and Washington, have aggressively used assisted living and other residential care options as an alternative to nursing home care for their Medicaid beneficiaries and have been successful in either preventing such placement or in relocating nursing home residents to assisted living or adult foster homes (Stone and Reinhard 2007).

Adult Foster Care and Adult Family Care. This residential care option is a small group setting housing just a few residents. As of December 2008, 30 states reported that 18,901 adult foster care homes were operating with a capacity to serve approximately 65,000 residents (Mollica, Sims-Kastelein, Cheek et al. 2009). Twenty-nine states license or certify these facilities; 17 cover them under their assisted living regulations. The importance of creating a "home-like" atmosphere in community-based residential care settings—including a focus on private rooms and bathrooms—was a major impetus for the expansion of adult foster care in many states (Golant and Hyde 2008). This setting closely resembles a private home in the community. In the typical model, the owner of the home or someone hired by the owner lives there and provides the cooking, housekeeping, and personal care services that residents need. In many cases, the owner started out as a family caregiver and then opened up the home to a few other residents (Mollica, Booth, Gray et al. 2008).

In a five-state case study of adult foster care, Mollica and colleagues (2008) found that there is a lack of awareness of this option among many potential providers and consumers. They also found evidence of a decline in the availability of this residential alternative. In Arizona, for example, study respondents indicated that this decline was due to competition with other home and community-based options. On the other hand, respondents in Oregon and Washington identified inadequate Medicaid reimbursement rates as a deterrent to this option. The researchers noted that Wisconsin is exploring tax incentives as a way to expand its adult foster-home stock.

Independent Senior Housing Linked with Services. Approximately 1.3 million low-income elderly individuals live in publicly subsidized rental housing, including Section 202 housing for the elderly (263,000); other HUD–subsidized, private-owner, multifamily housing properties (422,000); public housing (305,000); and recipients of Section 8 housing choice vouchers (334,000) (Haley et al. 2008). An additional unknown number of elderly people live in rental properties subsidized by low-income housing tax credits (LIHTCs) restricted to or primarily for seniors.

Many of these elderly residents moved into publicly subsidized rental housing when they were in their 60s; a large segment of them have "aged in place," become disabled, and are in need of long-term care. The median age of residents in Section 202 properties and other multifamily subsidized senior properties is 74, and approximately a third of residents are age 80 and over (Haley et al. 2008). Several national surveys and small studies provide an indication of residents' functional status and, thus, their potential need for services and supports. Data from the 2002 American Community Survey indicate that over half of subsidized elderly renters reported limitations in such activities as walking and climbing stairs, and a third reported difficulty with shopping or going to the doctor (Gibler 2003). A 2006 survey conducted by AARP of Section 202 and LIHTC property managers found that 38 percent of elderly LIHTC residents were perceived to be frail and disabled (Kochera 2006). A recently completed survey of residents in four subsidized senior housing properties in the San Francisco Bay area with a large culturally diverse population and median age of 78 years old found that 36 percent reported two or more ADL limitations and 63 percent needed assistance with two or more ADLs; 35 percent reported a memory-related disease diagnosed by a doctor; 35 percent reported falling in the past year, with an average of 2.2 times; and 32 percent visited the emergency room one or more times during the year and 20 percent reported an overnight hospital stay (American Association of Homes and Services for the Aging 2010).

HUD's Congregate Housing Services Program (CHSP) offers grants to states, local government, public housing authorities, tribally designated housing entities, and local nonprofit housing sponsors to provide supportive services needed by frail elderly residents and residents with disabilities in federally subsidized housing. Today, 51 public housing agencies and private assisted housing owners administer programs that provide at least one daily hot meal in a group setting, service coordination, personal assistance, housekeeping, transportation, preventative health or wellness programs, and personal emergency response systems. A few states (Connecticut, Maryland, Massachusetts, and New Jersey) have also developed such programs. Across the country, some local senior housing providers have also implemented programs with their own resources or through partnerships with other organizations in their community to bring personal care, health services, and social services to their housing properties to help meet their residents' needs (Harahan, Sanders, and Stone 2006).

Adult Day Care

Another home and community-based setting is the adult day center. According to the most recent published data, there are more than 4,600 adult day service providers, a 35 percent increase since 2002, serving approximately 260,000 participants and family caregivers on any given day (MetLife National Study of Adult Day Services 2010). Adult day-services providers offer social activities, transportation (door-to-door service), meals and snacks, personal care, therapeutic activities (e.g., exercise, mental interaction), health monitoring, medication management, emergency respite, and caregiver support services.

There are two types of centers. The social model offers meals, recreation, and some health-related services. The medical or health model offers social activities, intensive health monitoring and oversight, and therapeutic activities. Some centers specialize in services for a particular population (e.g., individuals with dementia). Twenty-one percent of adult day centers are based on the medical model of care, 37 percent are based on the social model (with no or limited health-related services), and 42 percent are a combination of the two. There are no published data on the percent of centers that specialize in the care of a particular population.

Almost three-quarters (71 percent) of the centers are not-for-profit, and there has been some growth in for-profit providers from 22 percent in 2002 to 27 percent in 2010. About six out of ten centers operate under the umbrella of a larger parent organization, such as a home care agency, a skilled nursing facility, a medical center, or a multipurpose senior organization. Almost 80 percent of the centers have either a registered nurse or a licensed practical nurse on staff; about half of all centers (48 percent) employ social workers. Fifty-eight percent of the clients are women. Almost 7 out of 10 participants are age 65 and older, one in five are age 41 to 64 and the remainder are 40 years or younger. Approximately 4 out of 10 participants are nonwhite. A little less than half of center clients have some cognitive impairment.

Family caregivers are an important focus of adult day centers. Seven out of 10 organizations provide educational programs for caregivers, 58 percent sponsor support groups, 40 percent provide individual counseling, and 12 percent provide overnight respite care for families able to leave their disabled relative at the center to obtain temporary relief from their caregiving responsibilities.

The average capacity of an adult day center is 51 clients and the average staff ratio is six clients to one staff person. The majority of these programs are open Monday through Friday for eight hours; only a fraction have evening or weekend hours. With an average daily rate of $61 for 8 to 10 hours, many advocates for adult day care argue that this service can be very cost-effective, given that the average hourly rate for a home-health aide is $19. There have been very few outcome studies of adult day programs. One small study of adult day health-center enrollees in San

Francisco found an improvement in several quality-of-life measures over a one-year period compared with controls (Schmitt et al. 2010).

Conclusion

The long-term care system is a patchwork of providers and settings that offer individuals an array of choices. These choices, however, are constrained by how affordable and available the services are in a particular community. As chapter 4 will highlight, the family is the primary caregiver in most cases and often is the major navigator for the elderly individual who faces complex and often confusing decisions about how to obtain care in the most appropriate setting.

3

Who Needs and Uses Long-Term Care?

The elderly long-term care population is a heterogeneous group that varies demographically and receives services and supports in the range of settings described in chapter 2. This chapter provides an overview of this population and describes in more detail the characteristics and trends in both the nursing-home and home and community-based care populations. The chapter concludes with a discussion of the major factors that will influence future demand for long-term care as the baby boomers age over the next few decades.

Overview of the Long-Term Care Population

The long-term care population is diverse in terms of age and level of disability. Using data from the 2005 Survey of Income and Program Participation and the 2004 National Nursing Home Survey, Kaye, Harrington, and LaPlante (2010) estimated the size of the population using a broad and a narrow definition. Using the broadest definition—needing help with one or more ADLs or IADLS—they estimated that over 12 million people in the United States need long-term care at any one time. Approximately 10.9 million people of all ages (or about 4 percent of the community-dwelling U.S. population) are living in the community with long-term care services or supports. Half of the noninstitutionalized long-term care population is age 65 and older; the rest are under age 65. The broadly defined population living in nursing homes or other institutional settings is approximately 1.6 million people; 88 percent of that group is age 65 and older.

The more narrowly defined long-term care population includes people needing help with two or more ADLs. This group is of particular policy relevance because eligibility for many federal and state programs as well as long-term care insurance benefits are triggered by this level of need. The narrowly defined population includes 4.4 million Americans. Among the 3.1 million living in the community, 48 percent are under age 65. The vast majority of institutionalized people needing long-term care using the more narrow definition are age 65 and older. Only 11 percent are under age 65. As noted in chapter 1, the remainder of this chapter focuses on the elderly long-term care population.

Published estimates from the 2007 Medicare Current Beneficiary Survey indicate that community-dwelling elderly individuals living in residential care settings had greater long-term care needs as measured by their number of ADL and IADL limitations than those living in their own homes or apartments but fewer than those living in nursing homes (Federal Interagency Forum on Aging-Related Statistics 2010).

Table 3.1. Population Needing Long-Term Care Services in the United States by Age and Residential Setting, 2004–2005

| | AGE GROUP (MILLIONS OF PEOPLE) | | | | | | |
| | All Ages[a] | | Under 65 | | 65+ | | Percent under 65 |
	No.	%	No.	%	No.	%	
Community residents							
Broad definition[b]	10.9	4.1	5.5	2.8	5.4	15.5	50.2
Narrow definition[c]	3,1	1.2	1.5	0.6	1.6	4.8	47.6
Institutional residents							
Broad definition[b]	1.6	n.a.	0.28	n.a.	1.3	n.a.	18.2
Narrow definition[c]	1.3	n.a.	0.13	n.a.	1.1	n.a.	10.6

Sources: Kaye, Harrington, and LaPlante (2010).

n.a. = not applicable

a. Beginning at age 6 for Survey of Income and Program Participation.

b. Gets ADL/IADL help.

c. Gets help with two or more ADLs.

Figure 3.1. Percentage of Medicare Enrollees Age 65 and Over with Functional Limitations, by Residential Settings, 2007

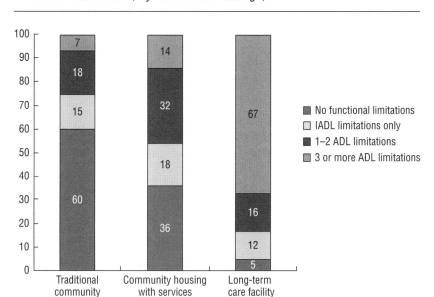

Source: Centers for Medicare Services. Medicare Current Beneficiary Survey.

Notes: Community housing with services applies to respondents who reported they lived in retirement communities or apartments, senior citizen housing, continuing care retirement facilities, assisted living facilities, staged living communities, board and care facilities or homes, and other similar situations, and who reported they had access to one or more of the following services through their place of residence: meal preparation; cleaning or housekeeping services; laundry services; help with medications.

Forty-six percent of elderly individuals living in community housing with services had at least one ADL limitation compared with 25 percent of traditional community-dwelling older adults. Among elderly nursing home residents, more than 8 in 10 had at least one ADL limitation, and 67 percent had three or more ADL limitations. As noted in chapter 1, long-term care needs increase with age. Among noninstitutionalized elderly individuals age 65 to 74, only 1.8 percent needed assistance with one to two ADLs. In contrast, among those age 80 and older, 8.2 percent needed assistance with one or two ADLs, and 10.9 percent required help with three or more ADLs.

On average, an estimated 69 percent of people turning age 65 in 2005 will need some long-term care over their remaining lifetimes, with an average duration of three years (Kemper, Komisar, and Alexcih 2005). Women have a greater likelihood than men of needing long-term care

Figure 3.2. Projected Lifetime Long-Term Care Needs for Persons Turning 65 in 2005, by Duration of Need

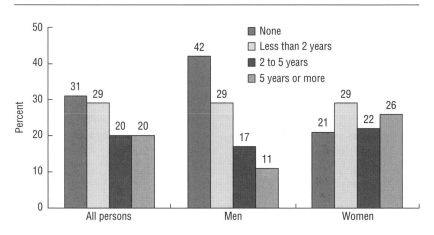

Source: Kemper et al. (2005).

after age 65 (79 percent for women and 58 percent for men). Thirty-five percent will use a nursing home, spending an average of nine months there. An estimated 13 percent will spend time in assisted living; 42 percent will use paid care at home, and 59 percent will get help from informal caregivers at home. One in five will need five or more years of care. These estimates, of course, could change dramatically if the nation experiences significant regulatory and reimbursement policy shifts that create incentives for more severely disabled older adults to receive services in other residential settings, including their own homes.

The Nursing Home Population

Analysis of the 2004 National Nursing Home Survey—the most recent data set to provide a cross-sectional view of the nursing home population in the United States—indicates that 1.3 million elderly Americans resided in nursing homes on any given day in 2004 (Houser 2007). Fourteen percent were 65 to 74 years old, 36 percent were 75 to 84 years old, and the remaining 50 percent were 85 years and older (Houser 2007). Comparative analyses of National Nursing Home Survey data from 1973 and 2004 indicate a continuing decline in the rate of use of nursing home care, particularly for the oldest old (Alexcih 2006).

Figure 3.3. Percent of Elderly Population Who Are Residents of Nursing Facilities

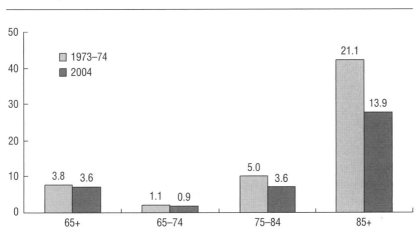

Source: Alexcih (2006).

A little more than one in five people age 85 years and older was in a nursing home in 1973, compared with a little less than 14 percent in 2004. The downward trends in age-adjusted disability rates are small and cannot account for the decline in nursing home use. Rather, the change is probably a function of the shifting configuration of available services, including

- a move toward short-term post-acute care being provided in nursing homes;
- an increase of Medicare home-health and home-care use; and
- the increased use of assisted living as a substitute for nursing home placement.

The nursing home population has become increasingly sicker and more disabled over time. Between 2004 and 2008, the proportion of nursing home residents with three or more ADL limitations increased from 49.8 to 57.7 percent (CMS 2009). Kasper and O'Malley (2007) compared data from the 1999 and 2004 National Nursing Home Surveys to examine trends in the long-stay population—those residing in a nursing home for at least 90 days and considered to be the "traditional" nursing home users (in contrast to the short-stay, post-acute care population). In 2004,

40 percent of long-stay residents had both physical and mental or cognitive conditions, compared to 25 percent in 1999. The percentage of
long-stay residents who received hands-on assistance with five ADLs
climbed from 26 percent in 1999 to 34 percent in 2004. This figure dou-
bles to 54 percent if supervision is considered as well.

While nursing home use rates have been declining since 1985, the
racial and ethnic composition of the national population of nursing home
residents has begun to shift. Between 2000 and 2005, there was a decline in
the percentage of nursing home residents who were non-Hispanic and a
slight increase in the percentage who were black or Hispanic (Alexcih
2006). The percentage of Hispanic residents increased by 1.4 percentage
points from 5 percent in 2000 to 6.4 percent in 2005; the comparable
estimates for black residents in 2000 and 2005 were 10 and 11.2 percent,
respectively. The for-profit providers were more likely than their non-
profit or government counterparts to have black and Hispanic residents.

There is evidence of racial segregation in nursing homes and a relationship between this segregation and the likelihood of residing in
poor-performing nursing homes. Smith and colleagues (2007) analyzed calendar year 2000 information from the Online Survey Certification and Reporting System and the nationally reported nursing home
Minimum Data Set (see chapter 7 for a more detailed discussion of these
reporting systems) to examine the relationship between the segregation
of whites and blacks and disparities in nursing home quality. They found
that nursing homes are relatively segregated, mirroring the residential
segregation within metropolitan areas. As a result, blacks are much more
likely than whites to be in nursing homes that have serious deficiencies,
lower staff ratios, and greater financial vulnerability. Black nursing home
residents were 1.7 times more likely than white nursing home residents
to be in a facility that was subsequently terminated from Medicare and
Medicaid participation. A similar analysis examining white and Hispanic
segregation in nursing homes found the same pattern (Fennel et al. 2010).

The Medicare Home Health Population

As noted in chapter 2, an important subset of the home-based population is the group that receives Medicare-funded home health services.
Findings from an analysis of 6.5 million episodes of home health care
ending in 2004 and 2005 indicate that 86.5 percent of the admissions
were people age 65 and over (Murtaugh et al. 2009). The largest share

(38.8 percent) was provided to people age 75 to 85 with a little over one in five of all episodes provided to people age 85 and over. Three-quarters of the care episodes were provided to people with one or more chronic conditions; a quarter were provided to patients with two or more chronic conditions, and 17.1 percent to patients with three or more chronic conditions. Home-health patients were assessed as being cognitively impaired in 36.2 percent of episodes. Further analyses indicated that both multiple chronic conditions and cognitive impairment are associated with longer home-health stays, suggesting that clinically complex elderly patients with both post-acute and long-term care needs present care planning and management challenges.

The Community-Dwelling Population

Approximately 80 percent of the elderly with long-term care needs live in the community (Kaye et al. 2010). As noted above, they tend to be much less disabled than those in nursing homes. Sixty percent are disabled only in IADLs. A little more than one in five are considered severely disabled, with limitations in three or more ADLs, compared with over two-thirds of the elderly nursing home population (Administration on Aging [AoA] 2009). As noted previously, level of disability increases significantly with age. Almost 42 percent of elderly noninstitutionalized adults with severe disability are at least 85 years old, compared with just 22 percent of older adults with no disabilities. Nearly 6 in 10 older disabled adults are not married, leaving them potentially vulnerable to the lack of live-in support. Widowed older adults make up over 47 percent of the severely disabled elderly population, compared with just 27 percent of their nondisabled peers (AoA 2009).

A published analysis of data from the 2002 Health and Retirement Study provides greater detail about the elderly long-term care population living in the community (Johnson and Wiener 2006). In 2002, 35 percent of older adults with severe disabilities and over 57 percent of unmarried older adults with severe disabilities lived alone. These individuals face special challenges because to the extent that they have family members to provide care, these caregivers are often not immediately available when emergencies arise. At the same time, most community-dwelling frail older people—9 in 10 older adults with long-term care needs—have surviving adult children, with a little over 62 percent having at least one child living within 10 miles. Despite the image of a very mobile

America, these data indicate that most disabled elders have some family members living close by and potentially available to provide care.

There is a strong relationship between educational attainment and disability. Nearly a third of those with severe disabilities did not complete high school and nearly a third never attended high school. In contrast, less than a quarter of those without disabilities lacked a high school diploma and only about one in 10 had no high school education.

Older adults with disabilities also have less income on average than those without disabilities (Johnson and Wiener 2006). For example, median household income in 2001 totaled $30,264 among those with no disabilities, $18,480 for those with moderate disabilities, and $14,160 among those with severe disabilities.

Consistent with their lower incomes, frail older adults have significantly less wealth than their nondisabled peers, and most of their limited assets are tied up in their homes. In 2002, median household wealth among elderly people with severe disabilities totaled $47,913, nearly three-quarters of which represented the value of their homes net outstanding mortgage debt. In contrast, most elderly people without long-term care needs have accumulated substantial wealth, with the median household assets totaling $205,869 for this group.

Figure 3.4. Household Income of the Noninstitutionalized Older Population, by Disability Status, 2001

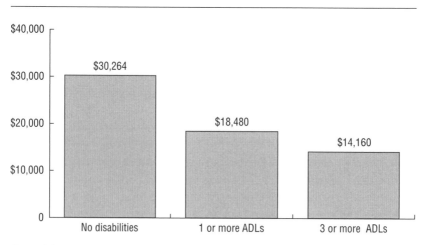

Source: Johnson and Wiener (2006).

Figure 3.5. Household Wealth of the Noninstitutionalized Older Population, by Disability Status, 2002

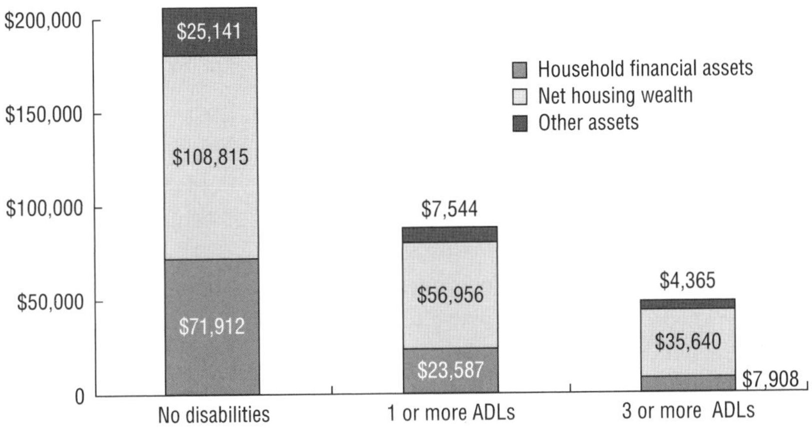

Source: Johnson and Wiener (2006).

Use of Assistive Technology

The definition of long-term care includes the use of assistive technology and special equipment, such as canes, walkers, and grab bars. Analyses of data from the Medicare Current Beneficiary Survey from 1992 to 2007 indicate an increase in the use of special equipment that help elderly disabled people with one or more ADL limitations to live independently in the community. In 1992, 49 percent used equipment and some personal assistance; 28 percent used special equipment only. In 2007, the percent of elderly disabled people using a combination of personal assistance and special equipment had increased to 50 percent; 38 percent used special equipment only to help them with their ADLs. This increase over time suggests that assistive technology is playing a larger role in meeting long-term care needs and helps mitigate the need for human assistance.

Unmet Need for Long-Term Care

Older people with disabilities who do not receive all the assistance they need with essential activities, such as bathing, dressing and cooking, face daily challenges in doing simple things that people without disabilities take for granted. If their needs remain unmet, they are at risk for more severe disability, hospitalization, and institutionalization.

Most of the literature on the magnitude of unmet need is seriously out of date. A 1997 review of the literature (Williams, Lyons, and Rowland 1997) found that estimates ranged from 2 percent to over 35 percent of community dwelling older adults with some unmet need, depending on what is included or excluded from the definition. Desai and colleagues (2001) analyzed cross-sectional data from the 1994 National Health Interview Survey's Supplement on Aging to examine the prevalence, correlates, and negative consequences of unmet need for personal assistance with ADLs among noninstitutionalized people age 70 years and older. They found that one out of five individuals needing help to perform one or more ADLs reported receiving inadequate assistance; the prevalence of unmet need ranged from a low of 10.2 percent among those with eating limitations to 20.1 percent with transferring limitations. Nearly half of those with unmet needs reported experiencing a negative consequence (e.g., being unable to eat when hungry) as a result of their unmet need.

A 2005 telephone survey of a random sample of people age 50 or older with difficulties in one or more of three activities found that almost 3 out of 10 respondents reported having unmet needs (Gibson and Verma 2006). Among this group, 37 percent received no help and the remainder received insufficient help. The primary reason cited for not receiving enough help was that the individuals could not afford assistance. Individuals who were eligible for both Medicare and Medicaid ("dual eligibles") were the least likely to report unmet needs. In addition, those living with and receiving unpaid help from a family member or other informal caregiver were less likely to report unmet needs. These findings underscore the importance of the Medicaid program as a safety net but also raise concerns about modest-income individuals who cannot afford to pay for services but have too many financial resources to qualify for Medicaid. The study also highlights a vulnerable long-term care subpopulation—those living alone without any family support to provide personal assistance services.

The Future Demand for Formal Long-Term Care Services

Several factors will influence the future demand for long-term care. These include the aging of the population, disability rate projections, the availability of family caregivers, the financial status of future cohorts of elderly individuals, and the ethnic and racial composition of this population in the future.

The Aging of the Population

As noted in chapter 1, the population age 65 and over is expected to increase substantially between now and 2030. But it is the growth in the 85 and older population—the group most likely to need long-term care—that will drive the demand for services. This growth is expected to accelerate between 2030 and 2050 to 21 million people by 2050 (Vincent and Velkoff 2010).

Disability Rates

As noted in chapter 1, the aging of the population is a key factor in understanding the current and future demand for services because of the strong relationship between age and the likelihood of being disabled. Future demand for long-term care services depends, in large part, on whether disability rates rise or fall. There is a growing consensus that limitations in IADLs and functional limitations, such as difficulty bending, reaching, and stooping, declined during the 1990s (Freedman, Martin, and Schoeni 2002). There is less agreement, however, about recent trends in the more severe type of disability that involves ADL limitations. One study found that the combined age-adjusted share of the older population with ADL disabilities or living in institutions fell by about 20 percent between 1982 and 2005 (Manton, Gu, and Lamb 2006). Other studies, however, have found no significant change in ADL disability rates (Schoeni, Freedman, and Wallace 2001) or even small increases (Crimmins and Saito 2000).

The fact that disability rates declined in the past, however, does not guarantee that they will decline in the future. Much of the recent decline in disability appears to be related to educational gains among older Americans (Freedman and Martin 1999). Average schooling levels will continue to rise in the older population (Smith 2000), but it is not certain that the strong negative relationship between education and disability will persist. Disability associated with the rising prevalence of diabetes and obesity in the younger population might offset the future decline in disability rates at older ages (Lakdawalla, Bhattacharya, and Goldman 2004). In addition, recent research found that adults born between 1948 and 1953 reported worse health in 2004, when they were age 51 to 56, than those born 12 years earlier reported in 1992, when they were the same age (Soldo et al. 2006).

Availability of Informal Caregivers

Given the pivotal role that family members—particularly adult daughters—play in providing care (see chapter 5), the availability of family caregivers will affect the future demand for formal services. The availability of family caregivers may decline over time because of rising divorce rates, increasing childlessness, and declining family sizes (Wolf 2001). Women born between 1956 and 1960 had only 1.9 children on average, compared with 3.2 children for women born between 1931 and 1935 (Redfoot and Pandya 2002). The share of women age 40 to 44 without any children almost doubled (to 19 percent) between 1980 and 1998 (Bachu and O'Connell 2001). The rising labor force participation of women may also reduce their ability to provide informal care. From 1980 to 2001, the labor force participation of married women age 45 to 64 increased from 47 to 66 percent (U.S. Census Bureau 2003).

Female life expectancy has long exceeded male life expectancy. While that trend is projected to continue over the next four decades, the gap between the number of women and men is expected to narrow (Vincent and Velkoff 2010). This narrowing is due to the more rapid increase in life expectancy in men that is projected over the next several decades. In 2010, for people 65 and older, the number of men per one hundred was 75.4. That number is expected to increase to 81.1 in 2030 and 82.1 in 2050. This narrowing is projected to be most dramatic for the "oldest old."

These trends have important consequences for the demand for formal services and the costs of public programs. If fewer family caregivers are available, many older adults may turn to paid services (assuming they can afford to purchase them). On the other hand, greater longevity by men may result in more married couples that will reduce demand for paid long-term care (Lakdawalla and Philipson 2002). Findings from an analysis of the Study of Assets and Health Dynamics among the Oldest Old (AHEAD) indicated that frequent help from children with basic personal care reduced the likelihood of nursing home use over a two-year period by about 60 percent for disabled elderly people age 70 and older (Lo Sasso and Johnson 2002). Thus, the reduced availability of informal caregivers may increase the demand for nursing home care. Similarly, in a study of determinants of home care use, frail older people with high-earning children received less unpaid care from their offspring and more care from paid sources than frail elderly individuals whose children had worse labor market prospects (Johnson, Toohey, and Wiener 2007). These findings imply that the demand for formal services is likely to rise in the future as the opportunity costs of care from adult children grow.

Financial Status

Individuals with greater financial resources are more likely to pay for services in the private market. The growth in the private, assisted-living market and the concomitant drop in nursing home rates, particularly among white elderly individuals, illustrate the role that resources play in consumer choice. As noted in an earlier chapter, most individuals prefer home and community-based options and those with the financial resources are more likely than less financially advantaged individuals to purchase services in the home or in some other residential alternative to the nursing home.

The economic status of future cohorts of elderly individuals will have a significant impact on the demand for formal services in the private market. In 2008, the elderly were substantially better off financially than younger adults or children (Bin Wu 2010). At the same time, among individuals age 80 and over—the likeliest candidates for long-term care—11.5 percent were poor, 19.6 percent had incomes below 125 percent of the federal poverty level, and 45.4 percent had incomes below 200 percent of the poverty level. And, as indicated above, those with lower incomes had most of their wealth tied up in their homes.

While the baby boomers as a group are more highly educated than comparable age cohorts in the past and were expected to be more financially secure (Redfoot and Pandya 2002), the 2008 recession raised serious concerns about the financial capacity of future cohorts of the elderly to afford long-term care. A study examining income and poverty among the older population (Bin Wu 2010) found that the median family income in the United States declined between 2007 and 2008, coinciding with the recession. The decline was greatest for households and families headed by persons age 45 to 54. After adjusting for inflation, median household income for this group was lower than it was in 2000. Although it is impossible to predict what this decline will mean for the financial status of the baby boomers as they age, it underscores the uncertainty about the demand for formal services in the future.

Ethnic and Racial Variation

The elderly population is projected to increase substantially in its racial and ethnic diversity over the next four decades (Vincent and Velkoff 2010). The elderly population is projected to be 42 percent minority in 2050, up from 20 percent in 2010. Among the 85 and over group, one out of three is projected to be minority in 2050, up from 15 percent in 2010. The proportion of the elderly population that is Hispanic is projected to increase quickly over the next four decades. In 2050, 20 percent of the population age 65 and over is projected to be Hispanic, up from 7 percent in 2010. The proportion of the oldest-old population that is Hispanic is also projected to increase by about 10 percentage points between 2010 and 2050.

This growing racial and ethnic diversity of the older population has implications for meeting long-term care needs and preferences, defining the role of paid and unpaid caregivers, providing services with cultural sensitivity, and training the paid workforce in cultural competence to meet these diverse needs. Today, black and Hispanic elderly people use less formal long-term care services than their non-Hispanic, white counterparts, but both have a greater rate of disability (Fennell et al. 2010). Given the fact that both groups have lower median household incomes and less wealth than their non-Hispanic, white peers (Alexcih 2006), they will likely have fewer resources available to pay for services in the future. They are, therefore, more likely to depend on informal care, Medicaid, or other public programs or to go without services. The evidence of racial segregation for both black and Hispanic elderly nursing home residents and its relationship to poorer quality in nursing homes also raises serious access questions for these populations.

The Size of the Future Elderly Long-Term Care Population

Taking these various factors into account, several researchers have projected the growth in the elderly long-term care population over the next three to four decades. Using the Urban Institute's dynamic microsimulation model of the elderly population (DYNASIM3), Johnson, Toohey, and Wiener (2007) developed three different disability scenarios. The intermediate disability scenario, which provides the "best guess" of the future size of the disabled elderly population, shows that between

2000 and 2040, the size of the elderly Americans needing long-term care will more than double, from 10 million to about 21 million people. The Lewin Group (2010), using its Long-Term Care Financing Model, projects that the long-term care population will grow from 6.2 million in 2000 to 15 million in 2040 and 16.1 million in 2050. Regardless of the estimate, the demand for formal services will clearly increase in the future. The next three chapters address the questions about how we will pay for these services, who will provide them, and how they will be delivered.

4

Who Pays for Long-Term Care?

Today, the financing of long-term care services is a patchwork of funds from federal, state, and local levels and private dollars. In 2008, national spending on long-term care for people of all ages totaled $243 billion; approximately $182 billion was spent on the elderly (The Lewin Group 2010). That figure is projected to nearly double by 2030 to $341 billion and to grow to $684 billion when all baby boomers have reached age 85 and over.

As noted in chapter 1, the costs of nursing home care and assisted living are out of reach for most elderly Americans and their families. For those with extensive home care needs, purchasing services is often not an option. The median annual private pay rate for homemaker or companion services in 2010 was $42,184; the comparable rate for a home health aide was $43,472 (Genworth Financial 2010). Among those paying out of pocket, the median monthly expenditure for home and community-based services from 2005 to 2006 was $280; the comparable estimate for nursing home expenditures in 2004 was $980 (Kaye, Harrington, and LaPlante 2010). Among persons turning age 65 in 2005 who will have out-of-pocket costs for long-term care during their lifetimes, 36 percent will have expenditures that exceed $25,000 and 10 percent will have expenditures that exceed $100,000 (Kemper, Komisar, and Alexcih 2005).

In 2008, public funds, primarily Medicaid and Medicare, accounted for approximately 74 percent of all national long-term care spending (including spending on the nonelderly population). Medicaid finances the majority of formal long-term care use (49 percent), Medicare pays for 22 percent, and other public sources finance 3 percent. Eighteen percent is paid for out of pocket and 9 percent is paid for by other private sources, including long-term care insurance.

These estimates do not include the dollar value of the vast amount of unpaid care, including the value of wages informal caregivers forgo. AARP estimated the economic value of this care (including family care provided to the nonelderly long-term care population) at approximately $375 billion in 2007 (Gibson and Houser 2008).

Concerns about affordability and the fraying of the safety net at both the individual and societal levels are driving the long-term care policy focus on financing services and supports (Stevenson 2008). Family caregivers strain under considerable burdens, caring for more chronically disabled—both physically and cognitively—and medically complex elderly relatives. Americans enter retirement with modest savings, uncertain

Figure 4.1. Total Long-Term Care Expenditures for All Age Groups by Source, 2008 ($ billions)

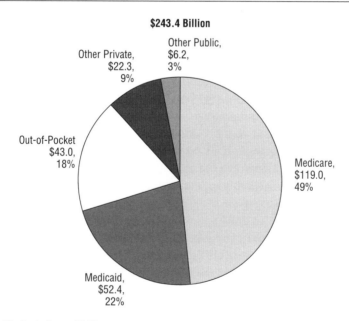

Source: The Lewin Group (2010).

about how they will afford routine costs of living, let alone catastrophic long-term care costs.

Over the coming decades, entitlement spending for Medicare- and Medicaid-funded long-term care is expected to absorb larger shares of federal revenue and threatens to crowd out other spending as the baby boom generation enters retirement (Allen 2005). Long-term care spending constitutes a substantial portion of Medicaid budgets—a third on average and ranging from 23 to 61 percent (The Lewin Group 2010). The increasing demand for long-term care services is already straining state budgets, a problem only expected to worsen over time. Because most states operate under laws that require an annually balanced budget—meaning that all spending must be fully financed—states must either cut other programs or reduce Medicaid eligibility, benefits, or provider rates. Without fundamental financing changes, Medicaid can be expected to remain one of the largest funding sources, continuing to strain federal and state budgets.

Policymakers, providers, and consumers are struggling with some fundamental issues with respect to the future of long-term care financing. These include determining societal responsibilities for meeting the demand for services and supports, assessing the balance of state and federal responsibilities to ensure adequate and equitable satisfaction of needs, determining the relative roles of the public and private sector in paying for long-term care (including the role of unpaid family care), and understanding the tradeoffs and consequences of these decisions.

Sources of Long-Term Care Financing

These policy questions set the framework for examining the current and future landscape of long-term care financing. The remainder of this chapter describes the various public and private sources of financing for long-term care. The chapter concludes with a discussion of the range of financing options being explored and the strengths and weaknesses each approach brings to solving the financing puzzle.

Medicaid

Medicaid is the nation's largest source of financing for long-term care. This jointly federal-state funded, state-administered health insurance program for the poor is required to provide coverage for nursing home care for elderly and disabled people who meet financial eligibility requirements (low incomes and negligible assets). Federal spending makes up slightly more than half the program costs. States pay a portion of all Medicaid costs and receive matching federal funds. Matching rates are determined at the state level and varied from 50 to 75.7 percent in fiscal year 2010 (Alliance for Quality Nursing Home Care 2010). In 2007, nursing home care accounted for 73 percent of total Medicaid spending on long-term care for elderly individuals and younger people with physical disabilities (Houser, Fox-Grage and Gibson 2009).

Since 1970, states have been required to cover home health services for those eligible for Medicaid-covered nursing home care and, beginning in the mid-1970s, states have had the option to offer personal care services under their Medicaid state plans (Ng, Harrington, and O'Malley Watts 2009). In 1981, Congress authorized the waiver of certain federal requirements to enable a state to provide home and community services (other than room and board) to individuals who would otherwise require skilled nursing facility (nursing home) services reimbursable by Medicaid. Waiver

Figure 4.2. Medicaid Long-Term Care Spending for Older People and Adults with Physical Disabilities in the United States, 2007 (percent)

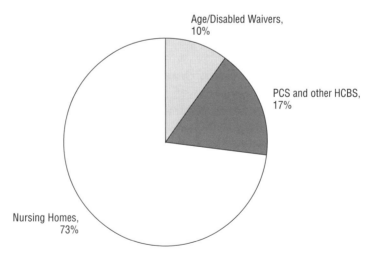

Age/Disabled Waivers, 10%

PCS and other HCBS, 17%

Nursing Homes, 73%

Source: Houser, Fox-Grage, and Gibson (2009).

services include case management, homemaker, home health aide, personal care, adult day health, habilitation, and respite care.

Spending for Medicaid long-term care per elderly person varies widely across the states (Houser, Fox-Grage, and Gibson 2009). In 2005, for example, Alaska spent $63,932 per person served on nursing home care. At the other end of the spending spectrum, Arkansas's Medicaid nursing home expenditures per person served were $15,856. With respect to home and community-based services, New York out spent other states at $19,552 per person served. In contrast, Utah spent only $2,357 per person served. Some of this variation is attributable to differences in the federal share of Medicaid spending, prevalence of disability rates among the elderly, and other factors. State coverage and reimbursement policies, however, are the most important differentiating factors.

Medicaid spending on home and community-based services has increased significantly over the past two decades. From 1992 to 2005, expenditures for these services grew at a rate of 15 percent per year, more than double the rate of growth for the overall Medicaid long-term care expenditures (Fox-Grage, Coleman, and Freiman 2006). Medicaid policies, however, are still biased in favor of nursing home care despite the fact that people feel less positive about this setting than any other provider of health or long-term care (KFF 2007). In 2005, Oregon and New Mexico spent over two-thirds of their Medicaid long-term care dollars on home and community-based services. In contrast, Washington, D.C., and Mississippi spent less than 20 percent of their Medicaid long-term care dollars on these services (Fox-Grage, Coleman, and Freiman 2006). In 2006, only seven states spent 40 percent or more of their Medicaid long-term care dollars on home and community-based care (Kassner et al. 2008).

It was primarily advocates from the disability movement that pushed states to take advantage of the Medicaid waiver opportunities beginning in 1981. More recently, the U.S. Supreme Court's *Olmstead* decision (1999) required that people with disabilities have the option of receiving services in the least restrictive setting. The Centers for Medicare and Medicaid Services (CMS), which administers Medicaid at the federal level, made the waiver process very flexible and invested millions of dollars in Systems Change Grants to assist states in their balancing efforts. "Money Follows the Person" grants have been awarded to help states move people from institutions into the community setting of their choice. Many states also invest their own dollars in helping to strengthen the home and community-based infrastructure. (See chapter 6 for more details on rebalancing long-term care.)

Medicare

The federal Medicare program, providing health insurance to almost all people age 65 or older and some disabled people under age 65, financed 22 percent of national long-term care expenditures in 2008, including 16 percent of nursing home care and 27 percent of home health care (The Lewin Group 2010). Although Medicare was legislated primarily to pay for acute and primary care, the program provides limited coverage of skilled nursing facility and home health care services to Medicare enrollees who meet certain requirements. Medicare pays for the first 20 days, and in part for an additional 80 days, of care in a skilled nursing facility for individuals requiring post-acute services, including intensive rehabilitation, following a hospital stay of at least three days. Medicare also pays for home health care—skilled nursing, therapy, and social work and aide services—for individuals who are unable to leave their homes because of their health and who require intermittent skilled care.

An estimated 4.9 million (15 percent) of Medicare beneficiaries received short-term post-acute services out of the 32 million beneficiaries who used services in 2007 (Ng, Harrington, and Kitchener 2010). From 1999 to 2007, the total number of Medicare post-acute beneficiaries grew by 21 percent, while their expenditures increased by 75 percent. Over that same time period, Medicare nursing facility users increased by 32 percent and home health users by 15 percent. Medicare is paying for a growing portion of total public nursing home spending, increasing from 23 percent in 1999 to 32 percent in 2007. The Medicare portion of public spending on home health care remained steady over the eight years at about 80 percent.

Other Federal Financing

In addition to Medicare and Medicaid, several other federal programs support long-term care services for the elderly. Title III of the Older Americans Act (OAA), legislated in 1965, established a network of aging services providers in every state—administered by state units on aging (SUAs) and local area agencies on aging (AAAs)—and authorized funding for meal programs and other community-based services. Title VI of the OAA established a comparable service system for Native Americans in the United States. Unlike the Medicaid program, OAA funds are not means-tested; all elderly people age 60 and over are eligible for benefits, although most programs target services to those most in need.

In 2000, the reauthorization of the OAA included a new program—the National Family Caregiver Support Program—that provides funds to local aging services organizations ($155 million in FY 2003) to develop services and supports specifically for family members caring for elderly relatives. This program, whose funds are administered by state units on aging and local area agencies on aging, is the first national initiative to formally recognize family caregivers as part of the long-term care system. The funds are dispersed through a congressionally mandated formula based on a proportionate share of each state's population age 70 years and older. Services include information and referral, assistance in gaining access to supports, individual counseling and support groups, caregiver training, legal and financial consultation, home modifications, and respite care.

As of 2009, a decreasing proportion of the SUA budget in most states comes from OAA funding (NASUA 2009). On average, 30 percent of the SUA budget comes from the OAA and one in four SUAs report that OAA funding is 10 percent or less of their budget. Other sources of funding include state appropriations (all 50 states), foundations and private grants (23 states), targeted taxes that include a tobacco tax, or other targeted tax assessment (10 states), and state lotteries in New Jersey, Pennsylvania, and West Virginia.

The Department of Veterans Affairs (VA) also funds a range of long-term care services for elderly and nonelderly disabled veterans. On any given day, more than 35,000 veterans receive institutional long-term care in VA nursing homes. Veterans can also receive home-based primary care (see chapter 6), adult day health care, homemaker and home health services, home hospice care, and community residential care. In FY 2009, 59 percent of the VA's total extended care population received care in noninstitutional settings (U.S. Department of Veterans Affairs 2010).

State-Financed Programs

States spent 1.2 billion on Home and Community-Based Services (HCBS) in FY 2007 (Mollica, Simms-Kastelein, and Kassner 2009). When spending on state-funded programs is added to each state's Medicaid long-term care spending for older people (and younger adults with disabilities), the amount of public funds devoted to HCBS increases by 1.3 percentage points. While this overall increase is small, the impact can be dramatic for a particular state. For example, Indiana's CHOICE program nearly doubled the state's effort in FY 2006, from 5.5 to 10.7 percent.

In 2007, states reported operating 53 single-service programs. Forty states and the District of Columbia reported spending for 63 multiservice programs in 2007. General revenues are the most common source of financing; a few states (New Jersey, Pennsylvania, South Carolina, and West Virginia) relied on casino or lottery revenue. Nine states also reported that local funding, mostly from counties, is available for HCBS. Fifty-six of Ohio's 88 counties, for example, support senior services programs through county levies, which generate approximately $100 million. Forty-three of the 115 counties in Missouri have local senior tax levy funds that may pay for HCBS. The funds are governed by local senior tax levy boards that have full discretion on how the funds are allocated and targeted to specific programs or services.

Private Insurance

As noted above, private long-term care insurance financed only about 4 percent of the elderly population's long-term care in 2004. A long-term care insurance market has existed since the 1960s, but it is only since the mid-1980s that national insurance companies began developing and marketing policies nationwide. About 1.2 million policies were in force in 1990, compared with 8 million in 2009 (Stevenson et al. 2010). Most purchasers of long-term care insurance buy their policies directly through individual insurance sales agents. On average, purchasers select daily benefit amounts of about $145, a benefit period between three and five years, and policies that offer a comprehensive set of benefits (Tumlinson, Aguiar, and Watts 2009). About half of individual policies sold in 2006 include 5 percent compound inflation protection, with the percent increasing with the purchaser's income. A policy purchased in 2008 priced to reflect typical coverage decisions costs between $2,140 and $2,460 per year for a single 60-year-old. The comparable policy for a married couple ranges between $2,952 and $3,340.

Insurers are selling a growing number of policies through employers and other groups. Purchasers in this market tend to earn less and be younger than individual policy holders—41 years old on average. Unlike employer-sponsored health plans, individuals who purchase long-term care insurance through an employer usually pay 100 percent of the premium and, as long as they continue to pay premiums, remain covered under the policy regardless of where they are employed. Employers can also permit employees to purchase separate long-term care insurance policies for spouses or parents. In 2005, 29 percent of long-term care insurance policies in force were held through employer-based programs (America's Health Insurance Plans 2007). In 2002, the Office of Personnel Management (OPM) began to offer access to long-term care insurance (with no employer contribution) to all federal employees and their parents and federal retirees. Despite the fact that the federal program's features have produced considerably lower premiums than are available in the current individual market, the take-up rate for this product has been similar to the rate for other employers offering long-term care insurance.

A number of reasons have been offered for a lack in the growth of the private long-term care insurance market (Stevenson et al. 2010). One argument, supported by several studies, is that the product is not affordable to a broad cross-section of Americans (AHIP 2007; Wiener, Tilly, and Goldenson 2000). Another potential deterrent is that at current modal ages of purchase, around retirement, about a quarter of the population would be rejected by insurance companies under current underwriting criteria (Tumlinson, Aguiar, and O'Malley Watts 2009). These criteria exclude people with pre-existing conditions that have a relatively high probability of rendering individuals eligible for benefits by their becoming dependent in several ADLs or dependent on full-time supervision because of cognitive impairment. Younger purchasers could avoid exclusion through such underwriting but would pay premiums and freeze in place for a potentially long time (30 to 40 years) certain modes of care that exist at the time of purchase but may not be available when they need to use the benefits. The typical indemnity or reimbursement-of-cost approaches are somewhat inflexible. They would also risk the dissolution of the issuing insurer at some time in the future. Furthermore, even though individual premiums are stable, state regulators can allow insurers to increase premiums for all policyholders within a class of policies issued.

Many people do not value this product because they do not consider themselves to be at risk for needing long-term care nor do they believe that they are liable for the costs of care because government or some other health insurance will pick up the tab. A study comparing long-term care policy "buyers" and "nonbuyers" corroborate the views of many analysts who have examined this issue (LifePlans, Inc. 2007). The single most important reason for purchase cited by the sample of buyers was to protect assets. This finding suggests that the purchase of a long-term care policy may be part of a broader retirement strategy for many individuals. Among the nonbuyers, one half of the sample expressed concern about the uncertainty of products in the future—what the policy would actually pay for, what services would be available to be purchased, and what is the potential for rate increases. Brown and Finkelstein's (2008) simulation model analysis supports the notion that the availability of the Medicaid program could influence the decision by many who might otherwise buy a policy to not make the purchase.

In the Deficit Reduction Act of 2005, Congress promoted the Long-Term Care Partnership—state programs that allow people who purchase approved private insurance policies to qualify for Medicaid while retaining a higher level of assets than would otherwise be allowed. As of July 2009, 36 states had adopted a Partnership program and more than 100,000 policies were in force (Stevenson et al. 2010). Although it is too soon to evaluate the impact of these programs on market penetration or Medicaid program costs, the experience in four states that have had this program since the 1990s shows that the program has influenced the design of higher quality products. But improved policies have not meant an increased volume of purchases, particularly among people of modest means to whom the program is targeted (Ahlstrom et al. 2004). Most purchasers of Partnership policies have substantial assets—the majority of purchasers in California, Connecticut, and Indiana had more than $350,000 in assets. These individuals would never previously have qualified for Medicaid, resulting in greater expenditures. The Congressional Budget Office (2006) has estimated that on balance, enabling all states to offer Partnership arrangements would result in a small increase in Medicaid costs—$86 million over 10 years.

The Community Living Assistance Services and Supports (CLASS) Program

Recognizing the lack of a robust private insurance market, particularly for those who are already disabled and would be medically underwritten out of any policy, advocates for the elderly and younger people with disabilities worked aggressively to ensure that the CLASS program was included in the Affordable Care Act. This new federally administered, voluntary program for long-term care was designed to address many of the private insurance limitations (Justice 2010; National Academy on an Aging Society 2010). Unlike most private policies, no underwriting based on preexisting conditions can be used to prevent enrollment or to determine monthly premiums. To lessen the potential for adverse selection, enrollment is limited to people who work; retirees and people with disabilities who are not working cannot enroll (Wiener 2010). Program premiums are to be fully paid for by individual workers through payroll deductions. For employers who agree to administer payroll deductions, all workers will be enrolled automatically. Individuals retain the right to opt out at any point.

Premium amounts are to be set by the secretary of the Department of Health and Human Services (HHS) at a level to maintain program solvency. To qualify for benefits, individuals must have paid premiums for at least five years, have a disability expected to last at least 90 days, and meet the functional eligibility criteria established by secretary. To ensure maximum flexibility and consumer choice, a cash benefit is provided, with the amount varying by level of disability. The average benefit must be at least $50 per day (plus an annual inflation adjustment), based on the expected distribution of beneficiaries receiving the varying benefit levels. There are no lifetime or aggregate limits.

Each enrollee is assigned (as needed) an advocacy counselor who provides beneficiaries with information on ways to access the CLASS appeals system, assistance on annual recertification and notification systems, and other assistance required under HHS regulations. Beneficiaries also receive information and advice from an assistance counselor regarding access to and coordination of long-term services and supports, eligibility for other benefits and services, development of a services and supports plan, and decisionmaking on medical care and advance directives.

The law establishes the CLASS Independence Fund in the U.S. Treasury with the secretary of Treasury to serve as the managing trustee. The secretary of HHS is required to regularly consult with the Board of Trustees and the Advisory Council to ensure that enrollee premiums are adequate to ensure the financial solvency of the CLASS program over the short and long term. No taxpayer funds may be used for CLASS program benefits.

At the time of this writing, staff from HHS and the U.S. Department of Treasury were working on the implementation of the CLASS provisions. Concerns have been raised that have important implications for the long-term solvency of this program. The lack of underwriting and the voluntary nature of the program suggest the likelihood of substantial adverse selection—that is, the potential that high-risk individuals (those with disabilities or at risk of becoming disabled) are most likely to enroll. These program elements, in turn, are key factors in determining the premium levels that need to be set to ensure a sustainable program. If the premium levels are too high, there will be little incentive for younger, healthier working-age individuals to enroll in the program. The SCAN Foundation and Avalere Health's (2010) premium simulator estimates average premiums to be three times what the premiums would be for a mandatory program in which everyone participated. Adverse selection most dramatically increases premiums below a 6 percent participation rate assumption (Tumlinson, Ng, and Hammelman 2010). Active marketing, therefore, will be critical to the program's success (Wiener 2010). There are also substantial implementation issues, including the relationship between CLASS and Medicaid and who will assume responsibility for eligibility determination and benefit administration.

The Future of Long-Term Care Financing

After 30 years of debate about how to pay for long-term care, the solution in the United States remains a patchwork of public and private mechanisms that includes significant voluntary in-kind contributions from family caregivers. The basic debate over long-term care financing is primarily an argument over the relative merits of the private-versus public sector approaches and the balance between the two strategies (Komisar et al. 2009; Wiener 2009). Some argue that the primary responsibility for the care of elderly people and younger persons with disabilities belongs with individuals and their families and that government should act as a payer of last resort. Those advocating the opposite perspective believe that long-term care can be affordable if the risk is spread across the entire country, similar to the experiences of other countries, such as Germany, Japan, the Netherlands, and Sweden. Between these two extremes are mixed models with varying degrees of public and private responsibility.

Private Sector Strategies

Private sector strategies are appealing because they are in line with the American tradition of individual responsibility and because they may help to hold down public spending by preventing the middle class from spending down to Medicaid eligibility. Wiener (2009) identified two broad categories of private sector approaches. The first is *individual asset accumulation and use* and includes a range of options, such as individual saving for long-term care and the use of reverse mortgages. Given the low savings rate in the United States, the first option within the category is not a viable solution. Reverse mortgages—home equity loans that do not have to be paid off until the borrower dies or moves from the house—may be viable for some portion of the elderly who have substantial home equity. But the various fees, restrictions, and interest payments and the almost "sacred" nature of one's home have limited the use of this mechanism (Foote 2009). The significant drop in housing prices resulting from the 2008 recession do not bode well for the future of this strategy.

The second broad strategy is risk pooling through various forms of *private long-term care insurance.* The limited growth of the current individual and employer-sponsored markets and the reasons behind this lack of expansion were described earlier in this chapter. One option within the private insurance category involves the creation of a new product that would combine retirement and long-term care insurance. The purpose of combining a lifetime retirement annuity with disability insurance is to overcome current barriers to the purchase of both products that result from insurers' expectations of adverse selection. The strategy is to let one risk offset the other—disproportionately healthy buyers attracted by annuities balancing disproportionately unhealthy buyers of long-term care insurance—thereby making underwriting and conservative pricing unnecessary. The disadvantages of this approach include the fact that the products are complicated and difficult to understand. In addition, only small premium savings are achieved by combining products (Wiener 2009).

Expanding the Long-Term Care Safety Net

Another option is to strengthen the protection for low- and modest-income elderly and younger people with disabilities by expanding the Medicaid program. The Affordable Care Act includes several policy changes and initiatives designed to encourage the growth of home and community-based services (see chapter 6 for more details). These include an increase in the Federal Medicaid Assistance Payments (FMAP) to states interested in expanding their Medicaid home and community-based care benefits. The ACA creates a new Medicaid state plan option—Community First Choice—that enables states to offer community-based personal care or attendant services and supports to those beneficiaries meeting the state's criteria for nursing facility eligibility. States that choose this option will receive a 6 percentage point increase in their FMAP. States will be allowed to adopt the more generous institutional eligibility criterion of up to 300 percent of the income threshold for Supplemental Security Insurance (SSI) benefits, thereby equalizing access to personal care services and institutional care based on financial criteria. They can also use funds to cover the costs of community transition supports (e.g., rent and utility deposits, bedding, and basic kitchen supplies) for institutionalized individuals who meet the eligibility criteria and wish to return to the community (Shugarman 2010). Beginning in 2014, this law also equalizes the spousal protection from impoverishment between those whose spouse enters a nursing home and those who choose to receive Medicaid home and community-based services.

Augmenting Medicare Post-Acute Care Benefits

As was noted earlier in this chapter, Medicare pays for a substantial amount of post-acute care nursing home and home and community-based settings. During the 1990s, the Medicare home health benefit was used by many beneficiaries with largely long-term care needs, but this practice was abruptly ended with the passage of the Balanced Budget Act of 1997 (Wiener 2009). One strategy for expanding access to these services is to remove the homebound requirement for home health care, which would allow more people with long-term care needs to receive services. A strategy for expanding the post-acute benefit to people who need skilled nursing care in a nursing home would be to eliminate the three-day prior hospitalization requirement. Of course, both options would add to Medicare costs, an action not likely to be looked on favorably by policy-makers or consumers already concerned about this entitlement program.

Social Insurance Program for Long-Term Care

The social insurance approach is based on the premise that the private insurance market will likely remain beyond the reach of many who need or are at risk of needing long-term care and that a universal social insurance approach—similar to Medicare or Social Security—is the most efficient way to establish a public/private financing solution. Like other social insurance programs in the United States, these proposals would establish a basic foundation around which private insurance could be wrapped. One approach would be to create a comprehensive social insurance system like those established in Germany and Japan (Campbell, Ikegami, and Gibson 2010). Both programs have mandatory participation, ensuring that the risk is spread across the entire population. The German program—financed through premiums—provides benefits to people of all ages who meet certain disability criteria. The Japanese program—financed half by premiums and half by taxes—covers all people age 65 and over who meet the disability criteria and people age 40 to 64 who have age-related diseases. German beneficiaries may opt for a cash benefit; Japan's program is limited to agency-provided services.

Campbell and colleagues (2010) note that both programs have been popular with the general public and have been accepted as a normal component of social policy in both countries. During the development of the health care reform legislation in the United States in 2009, however, it became clear that there was no appetite in this country for a mandatory program. Ultimately, the Congress enacted the CLASS program—described above—as part of the Affordable Care Act. Set to become fully operational by 2014, its voluntary nature and the myriad issues surrounding implementation make the future success of this new endeavor uncertain.

Policymakers, providers, consumers, and researchers will be closely watching the implementation of CLASS over the next five years to see whether this voluntary insurance program will be attractive to a wide range of working age people who will need to pay the premiums on an ongoing basis to make CLASS financially viable. It will be interesting to see how the private insurance market evolves as CLASS becomes operational over the next decade. To the extent that CLASS attracts primarily an older working-age, higher risk population, private insurers will likely market to a younger, healthier population. Private insurers could also create wraparound products to enhance the relatively modest CLASS benefits.

The long-term effects of both CLASS and the Partnership Program on the demand for Medicaid-funded services remain to be seen. Medicaid will likely continue to play a major role in financing long-term care, as a safety net for those who need nursing home care and home and community-based services. The fiscal pressures on the states during severe economic downturns, however, raise serious concerns about the long-term viability of Medicaid to meet the increasing demand for services over the coming decades. A large part of the costs of long-term care, therefore, will undoubtedly fall on the shoulders of family caregivers and personal resources.

The most recent 2008 economic recession has raised concerns about the ability of current and future elderly cohorts to pay for their long-care needs. Anecdotal evidence suggests that retirees who were planning to supplement Social Security with income from 401(k) plans, IRAs, and other savings have lost significant financial resources and have little prospect of recouping their losses (AARP 2008). In a 2009 survey of 4,412 Americans age 51 and older participating in the Health and Retirement Study, researchers found that older Americans have weathered the financial crisis relatively well, although they expect to work longer than they did a year ago (University of Michigan 2009). The survey also found that nearly a quarter of older Americans reported a decline in the value of their home. Slightly less than half still have home mortgages, and about 7 percent of these reported that they owe more on their home than it is worth. Researchers from the Urban Institute have also reported that in 2008 the retirement account of the typical household age 50 and older held a balance of $89,300, not enough to replace one year's pre-retirement income. While the long-term consequences of this recession and the potential for other future economic downturns are unknown, it is clear that the issue of how best to finance long-term care will remain a challenge.

5

Who Provides Care?

As millions of baby boomers march toward older ages, there are increasing concerns about the capacity of the caregiving workforce to meet the demand for long-term care. Much long-term care, in contrast to more medically oriented services, is unpaid assistance provided by family and friends (Stone 2006a). This has been true in the past, and despite the persistent myth of family abandonment fostered by some policymakers, consumer advocates, and the media, it remains true today (Gonyea 2009). As noted in chapter 1, however, there are uncertainties about how willing and available family members will be to play their pivotal role in caring for disabled elders in the future. In addition, many long-term care policy officials, providers, worker and consumer organizations, and researchers agree that the formal long-term care workforce is already in crisis (Stone and Harahan 2010). The crisis is reflected in labor shortages, rapid staff turnover, the inability of many consumers to find willing providers outside their families, and grave concerns about the quality of the workforce and how that translates into quality of care (IOM 2008).

This chapter provides an overview of the current long-term care workforce, including family caregivers, the direct care workers who provide the bulk of formal care, and the professional staff who oversee, manage, and deliver agency- and facility-based long-term care to older adults. This is followed by a discussion of factors contributing to the workforce crisis and long-term trends that may worsen or ameliorate future challenges.

The chapter concludes by identifying employer practices, education and training strategies, and public policies that may help ensure the availability of a stable and competent long-term care workforce in the years ahead.

Informal Care

The major long-term care provider is the family and, to a lesser extent, other unpaid informal caregivers. Estimates of the size of the caregiver population vary depending on the data and definition used. Researchers at AARP estimated that between 30 million and 38 million adult caregivers (age 18 or older) provided an average of 21 hours of care per week, or 1,080 hours per year, to adults with one or more limitations in ADLs or IADLs in 2006 (Houser and Gibson 2008).

The overwhelming majority of noninstitutionalized elders with long-term care needs—about 90 percent—receive some assistance from relatives, friends, and neighbors. Almost 67 percent rely solely on unpaid help, primarily from wives and adult daughters. As disability increases, elders receive more informal care. Eighty-six percent of elders with three or more ADL limitations live with others and receive about 60 hours of informal care per week, supplemented by a little over 14 hours of paid assistance.

Most elderly people with long-term care needs have a primary caregiver who provides the bulk of the care and obtains and coordinates help from other, secondary caregivers, unpaid and paid (Wolff and Kasper 2006). Three out of four primary caregivers are women. Thirty-six percent are adult children, and 40 percent are spouses. Given that the average age of the informal caregiver is 60, most primary informal caregivers do not hold paying jobs. Among the 31 percent who are in the labor force, however, two-thirds work full-time. Employed caregivers provide fewer weekly hours of assistance than nonemployed caregivers, but they still invest, on average, 18 hours per week. Two-thirds of working caregivers report conflicts between jobs and caregiving that have caused them to rearrange their work schedules, work fewer paid hours, or take leaves of absence (usually unpaid) from work. Among employed adult child caregivers, almost half (48 percent) were going it alone without additional help from family members, friends, or paid help.

Although precisely estimating the economic value of informal caregiving is difficult, analysts using conservative assumptions about the size of the caregiver population and the cost of replacing services have valued the annual contribution of informal caregiving between $103 billion and $375 billion (Houser and Gibson 2008; Johnson and Wiener 2006). Studies have demonstrated the additional value of this informal care in reducing long-term care costs by preventing or delaying nursing home placement. One federally funded study found that over a two-year period, older adults who received frequent help with basic personal care from their children were about 6 percent less likely to enter a nursing home than those with less support (Lo Sasso and Johnson 2002). People who have family caregivers tend to have shorter hospital stays (Picone, Wilson, and Chou 2003) and lower home-health and nursing home expenditures (Van Houten and Norton 2008).

Families can derive satisfaction and personal gratification from caring for an elderly relative, but there is also ample evidence that these responsibilities take a toll on caregivers' physical and mental health. Many studies have found that, relative to their non-caregiving peers, caregivers are at increased risk for stress, insomnia, fatigue, depression, anxiety, and stress-related illnesses (Connell, Janevic, and Gallant 2001; Pinquart and Sorensen 2003; Schulz and Sherwood 2008).

The Formal Providers of Long-Term Care

There are three broad categories of personnel who provide direct care:

- **licensed personnel,** the vast majority of whom are employed by nursing homes, assisted living facilities, and home-health and personal-care agencies. They include nursing home and home-health agency administrators, physicians, nurse practitioners, registered nurses (RNs), and licensed practical and vocational nurses (LPNs/LVNs), as well as therapists and social workers;
- **facility and agency-based direct care workers,** including nurse aides, orderlies, and attendants, who are largely employed in nursing homes, and home-health, personal-care, and home-care aides who deliver care in the recipient's home as well as in adult day care centers,[1] senior centers, and other aging organizations; and
- **self-employed providers** who are hired directly by consumers and their families.

Long-Term Care Professional Staff

Physicians are formally involved in long-term care as nursing-home and home-health-agency medical directors, and as the individuals who are required to sign off on nursing home and home health care plans. Nursing homes reimbursed by Medicare or Medicaid are required to have a physician medical director who is responsible for overseeing the medical care of residents and for participating in the design of the residents' care plan. Assisted living facilities and home-health agencies are not required to have a medical director, although many do.

Research on the responsibilities of physicians in long-term care settings is largely lacking. A 1997 survey by the American Medical Association found that the vast majority of physicians (77 percent) did not treat nursing home patients (Levy et al. 2005). Findings from a 2003 study of nursing home medical directors found that 86 percent reported spending eight hours or less per week in a facility, and 62 percent reported visiting the facility once per week or less (U.S. Department of Health and Human Services 2003). Although no comparable data exist for the home-health arena, coordination and communication between physicians and home-health agencies has long been regarded as inadequate.

The failure to attract more physicians to long-term care settings is attributable to several factors. First, few physicians within or outside long-term care have training that prepares them to address the needs of frail, chronically ill, and disabled older adults. A 2005 survey of graduating medical students found that 25 percent did not feel well prepared to care for older adults in acute care settings, and 42 percent did not feel well prepared to care for older people in nursing homes (Rueben 2007). The number of doctors certified in geriatric medicine is declining, even though individuals over the age of 65 make up 50 percent of all visits to physicians and 36 percent of hospitalizations. A government study also found that lack of payment incentives; too much time that must be spent on non-reimbursable activities, such as phone calls from the nursing home and communicating with staff, families, and other providers; and concerns about obtaining liability coverage were obstacles (Levy et al. 2005).

Nursing home, assisted living, and home health administrators are responsible for staff supervision and management and compliance with federal and state regulations. The federal government requires states to license nursing home administrators, although there are no national standards. The credentialing of administrators in assisted living facilities, home-health agencies, and other home and community-based service agencies is left to the discretion of states.

There are no national data on the number of active, licensed administrators in long-term care settings, or where they work. The National Association of Boards of Examiners of Long-Term Care Administrators (NABE) estimates there are between 22,000 and 25,000 licensed nursing home administrators, of which 16,000 to 17,000 are currently employed in nursing homes. Licensing requirements across states are highly varied—some states only require a high school diploma and passing an exam. The number of individuals who take the nursing home administrator exam has declined by 40 percent since 1998, and pass rates have also fallen.[2]

A study of more than 400 nursing homes found an annual turnover rate among administrators of 43 percent. Turnover was associated with higher than average proportions of residents who were catheterized, had pressure ulcers, and were given psychotropic drugs and a higher than average number of quality care deficiencies (Castle 2001). Other studies (Singh and Schwab 2000; Castle 2006) also show low retention rates and a tendency of some administrators to frequently rotate positions. Low retention has been linked to job dissatisfaction, particularly with pay, coworkers, and work overload—perhaps an indicator of inadequate nursing home staffing (Castle 2001).

Barriers to recruitment and retention include inadequate job preparation, dissatisfaction with pay and coworkers and work overload, a lack of reciprocity in states with more rigorous requirements to honor licenses issued in other states, the requirement in most states that candidates for nursing home administrator jobs serve an unpaid "preceptorship," and the burden of being responsible for federal regulatory requirements (Lindner 2007).

Nurse practitioners (NPs) are registered nurses with advanced training who operate in an expanded nursing role. They are sometimes employed in nursing homes to conduct physical exams, make urgent care visits, prescribe medications, and provide preventive care. An estimated 78,500 NPs are licensed in the United States, of whom 2,000 are affiliated with nursing homes (BHP 2006). An unknown number of NPs are also employed by home-health agencies. About 3,400 NPs are certified in geriatrics, although the proportion of NPs specializing in this area appears to be declining (Center for California Health Workforce Studies 2005). Freestanding nursing homes in states with high Medicaid reimbursement rates and those in urban areas are most likely to employ NPs (Intrator et al. 2005).

A small body of evidence supports the value of NPs in long-term care. A study comparing nursing homes with and without NPs found fewer hospital admissions among the former, although residents' functioning, physical condition, or satisfaction did not seem to be affected (Garrard et al. 1990). A survey of physicians who are members of the American Medical Directors Association found that most respondents perceived NPs to be very effective in maintaining physician, resident, and family satisfaction in nursing homes (Rosenfeld et al. 2004). An evaluation of a quality-improvement nursing home model in Wisconsin underscored the important role of the NP in overseeing the clinical modules and assisting the nurses and direct care staff in how to use data in both care planning and quality improvement (Stone et al. 2002).

Registered nurses (RNs) are responsible for ensuring the quality of clinical care in long-term care settings, assessing health conditions, developing treatment plans, and supervising licensed practical (or vocational) nurses and paraprofessional staff. Most nursing home RNs hold administrative and supervisory positions. Federal law requires that the director of nursing in a skilled nursing facility be an RN. RNs employed in home health care assess the patient's home environment, care for and instruct patients and their families in self-care, and supervise home-health aides.

There are an estimated 2.9 million RNs in the United States, of whom 312,000 are employed in long-term care settings, usually in nursing homes and home-health agencies (Bureau of Labor Statistics 2010). While the number of nurses are far fewer in the long-term care sector than in the acute-care sector, the RNs—particularly in nursing homes—are more likely than their hospital-based peers to be in high-level management positions. All federally certified nursing homes are required to have a director of nursing who is a licensed RN.

The RN workforce is aging, and many are nearing retirement. Almost all RNs are white women, although a small but growing proportion are foreign born and foreign trained. Half of the 15,000 new nurses in 2004 who were trained and licensed in other countries were employed in long-term care settings, although some served as direct care workers while completing U.S. nurse licensing requirements (Redfoot and Houser 2005).

Shortages of RNs across the health and long-term care sectors are ubiquitous. RN shortages were reported by 86 percent of states in 2002 (Moore and Payne 2002), and a recent study by Buerhaus, Auerbach, and Staiger (2009) indicates that despite the current easing of the shortage due to the recent recession, the U.S. nursing shortage is projected to grow to 260,000 RNs by 2025. In addition to concerns about short-ages, nurse turnover—particularly in long-term care—is high. The 2008 American Health Care Association (AHCA) survey of nursing home staffing found an annual turnover rate among nursing directors of 18.1 and 42.8 percent for staff RNs; 7.9 percent of RN positions were vacant. Analysts project that 8,000 new licensed nurses are needed just to fill current vacancies (American Health Care Association 2010).

While turnover and vacancy rates among RNs employed by home-health agencies have not been systematically studied, the U.S. Government Accountability Office (GAO 2001) found a 21 percent turnover rate among home-health RNs in 2001. A study of home-health and hospice agencies in North Carolina found an average annual RN turnover rate of 29 percent in 2007 (North Carolina Institute of Medicine 2007).

Licensed practical/vocational nurses provide direct patient care, such as taking vital signs and administering medications. A much higher proportion of LPNs work in long-term care than do RNs. Of the estimated 760,000 active LPNs, about 297,000 work in long-term care settings, most often in nursing homes and other extended care facilities (Bureau of Labor Statistics 2010). Turnover among this group of nurses is high; the annual rate in 2007 was 50 percent (AHCA 2008).

LPNs have a shorter, less rigorous path to credentialing than RNs, typically taking 12 to 18 months to complete licensing requirements, in contrast to RNs, who undergo two to four years of formal preparation. While the LPN scope of practice is more limited than that of RNs, these nurses play a pivotal role in nursing homes. Anecdotal evidence suggests that, with the exception of the director of nursing, it is not unusual for LPNs to be the only nursing presence in a nursing home. According to a 2003 survey conducted by the National Council of State Boards of Nursing, more than 60 percent act as charge nurses or team leaders with responsibility for supervising and directing the care provided by paraprofessional staff (Smith and Crawford 2003).

Recruiting and retaining long-term care nurses is daunting. Nursing schools and community colleges appear to make little effort to encourage students to consider long-term care careers. Most students do not receive adequate exposure to long-term care settings as part of their clinical training. Only about one in four baccalaureate nursing programs require any coursework in geriatrics, and most curricula do not include information on long-term care practice. Nurses, furthermore, lack financial incentives to choose long-term care careers. For example, RNs who practice in nursing homes and home-health agencies make about $6,000 less per year than hospital-based RNs (Bureau of Labor Statistics 2006).

Career mobility and advancement opportunities are also lacking. Staff turnover, vacancies, and inadequately prepared direct-care workers add to the burden and stress of the job, exacerbated by the overwhelming paperwork requirements associated with government regulation. Many nurses, therefore, view the long-term care workplace as unappealing. For those who are employed in this sector, they often do not remain in the position for long.

Social workers who have completed specific course work and field work in aging (typically at the master's level) represent one of the fastest growing segments of the profession (NASW 2006). These workers address a broad array of problems uniquely facing elders and their families, including functional impairment, psychological problems or cognitive impairments, grief and loss, legal and ethical issues, and end of life concerns. Estimates of the number of professional social workers in long-term care settings range from 36,071 to 44,156 depending on the data source used, including the sampling strategy and definition of "social worker."

According to standards promulgated by the National Association of Social Workers in 2003, social workers in long-term care settings focus on the following areas:

- the social and emotional impact of physical or mental illness or disability,
- the preservation and enhancement of physical and social functioning,
- the promotion of the conditions essential to ensure maximum benefits from long-term health care services,
- the prevention of physical and mental illness and increased disability, and
- the promotion and maintenance of physical and mental health and an optimal quality of life.

Social workers in the nursing home and assisted living settings are often the primary contact with the families of newly admitted elderly residents as well as the mediators between residents and staff in times of crisis. They are also involved in transition planning, particularly discharges from hospitals to nursing homes or home-health care. A subset of individuals trained as social workers provide care management services to community-dwelling elderly individuals.

Physical therapists provide services that help restore functioning and improve mobility for people who need rehabilitation following hospital discharge. These services also help maintain functioning or prevent further deterioration for those with chronic physical and cognitive disabilities. Of the estimated 173,000 physical therapists in the United States in 2006, approximately 40 percent worked in some type of long-term care setting (Bureau of Labor Statistics 2010).

Occupational therapists, another important part of the long-term care workforce, help residents and clients improve their ability to perform activities of daily living. There are no data on the proportion of the estimated 99,000 occupational therapists in the United States who provide services to the elderly long-term care population.

Consultant pharmacists have been involved in long-term care since 1974, when Medicare first mandated drug regimen reviews in nursing homes (Levenson and Saffel 2007). The consultant pharmacist's role includes the provision of information and recommendations to physicians regarding medications, identification of improper use of medications or the prescription of incompatible medications, and collaboration with the medical director and other staff to develop proper protocols for response to adverse events. This role has become more important as the number of medications administered to chronically ill and disabled elderly residents has increased.

Direct-Care Workers: The Hands, Voice, and Face of Long-Term Care

Direct-care workers are the core of the long-term care system, responsible for helping frail and disabled older adults carry out the most intimate and basic activities of daily life, such as eating, bathing, dressing, and using the toilet. They represent the largest component of the long-term care workforce. These individuals—employed by facilities, home-health and home-care agencies, or self-employed—work in occupations that include **nurse aides** (orderlies and attendants), **home-health aides,** and **home-care/personal-care workers.**

Of the estimated 1.5 million nurse aides working in 2008, half worked in nursing homes with the remainder employed in other residential care settings (PHI 2010). Another 922,000 direct-care workers were home-health aides and 817,000 personal-care and home-care aides were employed in home and community-based settings. As is true with licensed nurses, direct-care workers are almost entirely women (90 percent). Nurse aides tend to be younger than those employed in home care. The average nurse aide is in her mid- to late thirties, while the mean age for home-care workers is 46 years. The percentage of home-care workers over age 65, furthermore, is three times that of aides in nursing homes. About half of nurse aides are employed full-time, while two-thirds of home-care workers are employed only part time.

In 2008, the median hourly wage of direct-care workers was $10.42, substantially below the $15.57 estimate for all workers in the United States (PHI 2010). Inflation-adjusted wages for these workers show that, over the past eight years, while nursing assistants have experienced a modest increase in their hourly wages to just over $9.00 (measured in 1999 dollars), real wages for home-health aides and personal-care aides have both declined and are under $8.00 an hour (Figure 5.1).

A government study found that almost 18 percent of nurse aides and 19 percent of home-care aides have family incomes below the federal poverty level, while only 8 percent of nurse aides in hospitals were similarly poor (Decker, Dollard, and Kraditor 2001). In 2008, 44 percent of all direct-care workers lived below 200 percent of the poverty level and

Figure 5.1. Direct-Care Workers' Median Wages, Adjusted for Inflation, 1999 and 2008

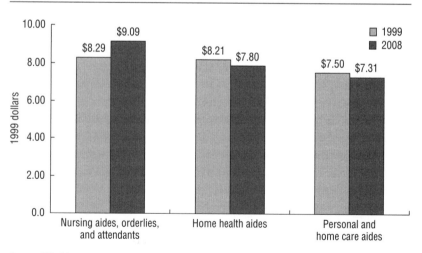

Source: PHI (2010).

two in five lived in households that were receiving two or more public benefits, such as Medicaid and food stamps (PHI 2010). Direct-care workers in long-term care settings—particularly those employed in home care—are also much less likely to have health insurance coverage than their peers in other jobs.

In 2007, an estimated 36 percent of home-health aides were uninsured; the comparable figures for certified nurse aides in nursing homes and hospitals were 23 and 11 percent, respectively (Figure 5.2). While two-thirds of Americans under age 65 receive health care coverage through an employer, only about half of direct-care workers (53 percent) have employer-based coverage. There are, furthermore, large disparities across settings. Only 36 percent of home-health workers report enrollment in employer-provided health insurance programs, compared with 58 percent of nursing home workers and 80 percent of direct-care workers in hospitals. Home health care workers are much more dependent on public coverage than their nursing home and hospital peers; roughly a fifth of home-care workers are enrolled in public plans, compared with 13 percent in nursing homes and 3 percent in hospitals.

The direct-care workforce is far more diverse than that of licensed nurses. A little more than one in five workers (23 percent) are foreign

Figure 5.2. Health Insurance Status of Direct-Care Workers (Percentage) by Setting, 2007

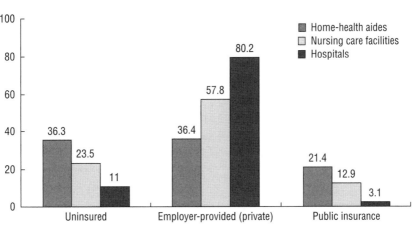

Source: 2007 National Survey of State Initiatives of the Direct-Care Workforce: Key Findings.

born, and many were educated in another country (Leutz 2007; PHI 2010). A third are African American, and 15 percent are either Hispanic or other workers of color. Nursing home aides are more likely to be African American and home-care workers are more likely to be Hispanic (Montgomery et al. 2005). As the workforce becomes more diverse, communication issues and the manner in which various cultures differ with respect to caregiving becomes more important. Results of the 2000 Census show that almost 12 percent of nurse aides in long-term care settings report they cannot speak English or speak it very well (Redfoot and Houser 2005). A recent study in four nursing homes found that Philippina LVNs were more uncomfortable than black or white nurses in carrying out supervisory responsibilities—or even raising issues to the director of nursing that might improve the workplace. Such assertiveness was not part of their cultural norms. The study also uncovered staff tension resulting from language and communication differences between racial and ethnic groups (Stone et al. 2007).

To become certified as a nurse aide, federal law requires less than two weeks of training or passing a certification exam, although most states add on to these requirements. Home-health aides must pass a federally mandated competency exam for their employers to receive reimbursement from Medicare. Federal continuing education requirements for home-health aides and nurse aides are minimal, and content is left to states and providers. The states determine the regulation of other direct-care workers, including those who work in assisted living, personal-care, and home-care agencies. Typically staff in these settings receive little or no training.

Self-employed home-care workers are hired directly by consumers to provide personal assistance services and other supportive tasks. Montgomery and colleagues (2005) estimate over 134,000 home-care workers are self-employed. Federal and state support of consumer-directed models of service delivery have stimulated the growth of self-employed home-care workers. Consumer-directed models enable care recipients to hire, direct, and fire their own home-care workers. In some states, these models also enable care recipients to employ family members to provide needed care. Studies find that when the opportunity is available, from 40 to almost 80 percent of participants in consumer-directed programs hire relatives to care for them. Job satisfaction and stress are equal to or more positive for consumer-directed workers than for those who work for an agency (Benjamin and Matthias 2004).

The evaluation of the federally sponsored Cash and Counseling Demonstration, which enabled disabled beneficiaries to hire and fire their personal assistance workers and pay them directly, found that the wages of consumer-directed workers were about 15 percent higher than agency-directed workers in two of the three demonstration states and 5 percent less in the other state. About 40 percent of consumer-directed workers said they were satisfied with their wages and benefits, in contrast to only about 20 percent of agency-directed workers. Injury rates across both groups were comparable (Dale et al. 2005).

Workforce Shortages and the Implications for Quality and Access

Perhaps the worst challenge to developing a quality long-term care work-force is the failure to attract and retain adequate numbers of high-quality direct-care workers to provide hands-on care. National estimates of turnover rates in the published literature are only available for nursing homes. The most recent data on turnover and vacancies from AHCA's 2008 nursing home staffing survey showed an annual turnover rate among certified nurse aides of 53.5 percent and a vacancy rate of 5.7 percent, a shortfall of about 43,700 workers (American Health Care Association 2010). In 25 states, the average turnover was above the 53.5 percent figure. Freestanding rural facilities had the highest turnover rates for direct-care workers. In 2007, furthermore, the perceived difficulty in recruiting nursing assistants was greater than the perceptions about problems with recruitment of RNs and LPNs (American Health Care Association 2008).

Recruiting and, more importantly, retaining a quality direct-care work-force have become major issues for providers, workers, consumers, and policymakers at the state and federal levels (Stone and Wiener 2001; Institute of Medicine 2008). Successful achievement of these goals is dependent on a variety of interdependent factors, including the value that society places on caregiving; local labor-market conditions, including wage levels and the degree of unemployment; long-term care regulatory and reimbursement policies; federal, state, and local workforce resources targeted to this sector; and immigration policy. The confluence of these factors and individual employer and employee decisions are played out in the workplace. Organizational philosophy and management style, wages and benefits, quality of the work environment, and interpersonal dynamics affect the successful development of the front-line workforce (Stone and Dawson 2008).

Impact of Workforce Shortages

A substantial body of research has addressed the relationship between turnover levels and quality of resident care in nursing homes, although much less attention has been paid to the relationship between quality outcomes and specific skills and behaviors. Studies of these relationships in other residential settings and home care are lacking.

A meta-analysis of the literature identified 87 articles and reports published between 1975 and 2003 that showed a direct relationship between higher nursing home staffing levels, particularly of licensed nursing staff, and improved quality of care (Bostick et al. 2006). This review also found a strong association between poorer resident outcomes and high turnover. High turnover rates in nursing homes have been associated with greater use of restraints, catheters, and psychotropic drugs; more contractures and pressure ulcers; and quality of care deficiencies reported on state surveys (Castle, Engberg, and Men 2007).

While there is a paucity of research on the link between quality and home and community-based workforce shortages, there is evidence that a shortage of direct-care workers in the home-care industry has an impact on consumer access to services. Evaluation results from the Cash and Counseling Demonstration program (see chapter 6 for a detailed description) found that participants who relied on the traditional agency-based service system were often not able to obtain the services because of worker shortages (Brown and Dale 2007). In their analysis of five years of data from the National Long-Term Care Survey, Spillman and Black (2005) found that the proportion of community-dwelling elderly care recipients who relied on formal care dropped from 43 percent in 1994 to 34 percent in 1999, while the proportion who relied entirely on informal care increased from 57 percent to almost 66 percent. While some of this reduction resulted from federal budget cuts in the Medicare program, the authors also attributed some of the reduction to a shortfall of paid home-care workers.

Factors Contributing to the Workforce Crisis

The Bureau of Labor Statistics projects substantial growth in the home-care and, to a lesser extent, the nursing home industry over the next decade (BLS 2010). With so many job openings anticipated and rising demand for services, shortages in the long-term care workforce seem to be at odds with classic economic theories of supply and demand. There are a number of reasons employers in long-term care settings are not able to compete effectively in the labor market.

Shrinking Labor Pool

The labor pool that has historically provided caregiving services to the long-term care population is shrinking at the same time that demand is increasing. Baby boomers had a smaller than average number of children than their parents. The native-born population age 25 to 34, from which both paid and informal long-term care providers largely come, will not increase at all between now and 2015. In addition, aging nurses are retiring and there is a serious shortage of young nurses to replace those leaving the field. Those entering the field, furthermore, are much more likely to be employed in the acute-care sector than to seek a job in the long-term care sector. As a consequence, long-term care employers cannot rely on traditional sources of labor.

Negative Image of Long-Term Care

Negative stereotyping of long-term care environments and workers discourages new job entrants. A Kaiser Commission Survey of public attitudes toward long-term care found that nursing homes rank below drug companies and just above health insurance companies in the share of adults who think they do a good job. Six in 10 respondents said they thought nursing homes make people worse off (KFF 2007). Ageism in the broader culture, the sensationalizing of nursing-home and assisted-living scandals in the media, and negative attitudes of educators and leaders in professional schools and associations conspire to reinforce the image of long-term care as a poor career choice. Among high school students considering a nursing career, for example, almost half have no interest in specializing in geriatrics, whereas 87 percent report having an interest in pediatric nursing (Evercare 2007).

Noncompetitive Compensation

Compensation and benefits for all staff categories are not competitive. For instance, compared with nurses in hospital settings, RNs who work in nursing homes or other extended-care facilities receive lower annual earnings on average, even though they work more hours per week, incur more overtime, and have a larger percentage of mandatory overtime hours (BHP 2006). Stakeholders in some states have observed that acute-care hospitals are able to draw staff away from long-term care employers by offering higher salaries or better benefits (Center for Health Workforce Studies 2005).

In 2007, *Forbes* magazine profiled personal and home-care aide jobs as one of the 25 worst-paying occupations in America.[3] In 2005, the average annual earnings of female direct-care workers were significantly lower than the average annual earnings of female workers in general ($17,228 versus $30,441), and 19 percent of female direct-care workers had incomes below the federal poverty level, versus 8 percent of female workers in general (Smith and Baughman 2007). Employers, furthermore, have a diminished capacity to increase wages because more than 70 percent of their financing comes from Medicaid and Medicare, which seek to limit costs regardless of labor market conditions.

Direct-care workers also have limited access to employee benefits, including health insurance coverage, sick leave, and retirement benefits (Smith and Baughman 2007; Stone and Dawson 2008). These workers are often unable to afford their share of health insurance premiums or they are ineligible for coverage because they work part time or work independently of an agency.

Challenging Work Environment

Workforce environments typically do not support front-line supervisors and direct-care workers, starting with a hierarchical chain of command that discourages involvement of lower-level staff in care planning and decisionmaking. Not surprisingly, LPNs, nursing assistants, and home-care aides do not feel that their jobs are respected, a perception that contributes to job dissatisfaction and high turnover rates (Bishop et al. 2008; Bowers, Esmond, and Jacobson 2003; Wiener et al. 2009). Other workforce challenges include inflexible work flow and job design, ethnic and racial tensions due to cultural diversity of staff and consumers in long-term care settings, and a paucity of career advancement opportunities (Wiener et al. 2009; Castle and Engberg 2006).

Caring for older adults can be physically taxing. Direct-care staff in nursing homes have one of the highest rates of workplace injury among all occupations. In 2006, the rate of nonfatal occupational injury and illness involving days away from work was 526 incidents per 10,000 workers among nursing aides, orderlies, and attendants (BLS 2007). This was four times the average rate among all occupations and was a higher rate than found among construction workers or truck drivers. Nursing aides, orderlies, and attendants also had the highest rate of musculoskeletal disorders among all occupations examined.

Inadequate System of Education and Training

The preparation of potential candidates for long-term care positions is out of sync with the realities of the long-term care demand and practice. Medical, nursing, and social work students have little exposure to long-term care in their curricula or clinical placements (Harahan and Stone 2009). Only a fraction of these students receive training in geriatrics, and even then, the focus is primarily on acute and primary care (IOM 2008; Stone and Harahan 2010). Administrators, nurses, and medical directors are poorly prepared for the management and supervisory roles with which they are charged in long-term care settings, and there are few in-service training programs to help those already employed in these positions (Bowers et al. 2003; IOM 2008; Harahan and Stone 2009).

The strategies regulators and educators employ to prepare and license or certify the workforce and to ensure personnel can keep pace with changes in clinical knowledge and new technologies are not effective. Relatively few standards or competencies are specific to long-term care. There is, furthermore, a huge shortfall of personnel who are competent in and committed to educating and preparing direct-care workers for long-term care careers. This translates into a dearth of people—both current and in the pipeline—who are adequately trained and educated to assume increasingly complex jobs across the long-term care settings.

This inadequacy of investment in education and training is compounded by the need for better knowledge and skills to respond to new philosophies and models of care. Emerging philosophies, such as person-centered care and culture change in nursing homes, have catalyzed the design of service delivery models that emphasize the role of the consumer and family members in decisionmaking and that empower lower-level staff to be more involved in managing the workplace and clients' decisions (Hamilton and Tesh 2002; Kane, Lum, et al. 2007). The growth in publicly funded programs that give the consumers the resources and the authority to hire and fire their workers—including their own family members—raises serious workforce issues. These include the magnitude and scope of training that should be required, and the roles and responsibilities that consumers can or must assume when they become employers (Foster et al. 2003).

With the expansion of home and community-based services, many states have changed their laws to allow nurses to delegate tasks to direct-care workers under their supervision (Reinhard et al. 2003). The implications of delegation for training and oversight in such areas as medication management and wound care are significant, leading the National Council of State Boards of Nursing and the American Nurses Association to call for the development of competencies and training programs for supervisory nurses to facilitate safe empowerment of direct-care workers (Harvath et al. 2008).

The increasingly complex health and functional needs of the elderly long-term care population also present training and education challenges. The presence of multiple chronic conditions and dementia in long-term care recipients exacerbates the already difficult problem of coordinating and managing transitions back and forth across settings: hospitals, nursing homes, assisted living, and home care (Coleman and Berenson 2004). It is difficult to see how the new chronic care management and transitional care demonstrations funded by the Affordable Care Act can be successfully implemented in light of the lack of trained, competent professional and direct-care staff to carry out the required roles and responsibilities. The growth in hospice programs in long-term care settings and the proliferation of palliative-care approaches to end-of-life services underscore the need for better formal and in-service training for all direct-care staff (Huskamp et al. 2010).

The trend toward more sophisticated information technology in care planning and coordination within and between care settings highlights another gap in educating and training staff. The success of health information technology in improving efficiency and quality is dependent on a competent, knowledgeable staff that understand how to operate the system and use the data. Most professional and direct care staff are currently not trained in how to use these data tools and systems.

Solutions to the Workforce Crisis

To meet the current and future long-term care demands of an aging society, policymakers, providers, educators, and other stakeholders must take action in three key areas.

Expand the Supply

Explicit policies must be developed to expand the supply of personnel entering the field. Today's developers of advanced training programs in geriatrics for professionals other than physicians must look to private foundations for support, or individual students must pay for the programs. IOM (2008) and Harahan and Stone (2009) identified several public policy strategies to help attract individuals into administrative and clinical professions in the long-term care sector. These include creating financial incentives, such as grant programs, to foster interest among people considering the long-term care field; scholarships, federal traineeships, and residency programs for people preparing for advanced degrees in long-term care; matching grants to fund administrator-in-training programs for people interested in management positions; and loan forgiveness programs for people who commit to long-term care careers.

The Affordable Care Act established a 15-member national commission to review projected workforce needs and recommend ways to align federal health care workforce resources to meet them (AAHSA 2010). Grants will be available for states to do comprehensive workforce planning and development. The health care reform also increased the loan amounts in the nursing student loan program and identified long-term care as one of the priority areas.

The U.S. Department of Labor's Long-Term Care Regional Apprenticeship program illustrates how targeted programs can be used as public policy tools to expand the supply of direct-care workers. Currently available in 20 states and in the process of being evaluated, this program combines classroom and on-the-job training with career advancement opportunities to expand the pool of nursing assistants and home-care aides (U.S. DOL/ETA, 2008). The public authority model—established in certain states (California, Washington) and localities (many counties in California) to support independently hired personal-care workers—could be used more extensively to recruit individuals into these direct-care jobs.

Older workers also provide a potentially rich pool of direct-care workers (Hwalek, Straub, and Kosniewski 2008). Research findings indicate that both older adults and long-term care providers are interested in exploring the potential of older workers and retirees to fill some of the current and future workforce gaps. Accordingly, several grantees of the Senior Community Service Employment Program, administered by the U.S. Department of Labor, have developed initiatives to train and employ lower-income older adults as direct-care workers.

Another potential pool of long-term care workers is the TANF recipient population. Recognizing this opportunity, the U.S. Department of Health and Human Services' Administration for Children and Families (ACF) recently announced a $51 million program, Health Profession Opportunity Grants, that will fund up to 17 five-year projects that provide training for and support educational paths to careers in health professions for TANF recipients and other low-income individuals (ACF 2010). Long-term care professions—including nursing assistants, home-care aides, and RNs—are specifically identified in the call for proposals. Projects must integrate the education and training with supportive services (e.g., transportation, dependent care, temporary housing) and must result in an employer- or industry-recognized certificate or degree.

Long-term care providers have also partnered with local high schools to develop on-site training and internship programs for students to attract them to careers in the field. These programs combine didactic, classroom education with on-the-job training, support from mentors, opportunities for communication with and shadowing of various long-term care staff, and the offer of jobs upon successful completion of the program.

Another important source of professional and frontline staff is the immigrant population. A recent study of the role of migrant workers in caring for the elderly reported that approximately one out of seven professional staff working in long-term care is foreign born; the comparable estimate for direct-care workers is one in five (Martin et al. 2009). Although many employers view immigrants as a valuable resource, there are impediments to this strategy as a solution to the pipeline problem. Immigrants may only come into the United States with a temporary or permanent visa. Visas for all temporary and permanent less-skilled workers are capped at 5,000 per year, making it almost impossible for long-term care employers to draw on them to recruit new personnel. Limits for higher-skilled personnel, such as nurses and physicians, are less restrictive (Leutz 2007). The future of immigration remains unknown, but the decisions made will have significant implications for the development of the long-term care workforce.

Invest in Workforce Education and Training

A high-quality workforce depends, in large part, on the investments that society makes in education and ongoing training of new and experienced personnel. The formal system of education, both initial and continuing, of long-term care managers, licensed professionals, and direct-care staff must undergo significant reform. Policymakers at the state and federal levels, educators, employers, workforce developers, and organizations representing the various occupational categories should jointly assess the adequacy of current educational efforts, including the extent to which these efforts specifically address the developmental needs of the long-term care workforce. Policymakers and other stakeholders should also evaluate the effectiveness of professional schools, community colleges, and other vendors in providing the education. Based on these assessments, they should determine the curricula and the competencies necessary to strengthen and expand the long-term care workforce—with a particular focus on how care should be delivered in emerging home and community-based care settings and through new service delivery approaches (e.g., transitional care, integrated care, consumer direction). Financial incentives should be made available to recruit and develop qualified faculty who have the skills and knowledge and are committed to educating and preparing long-term care managers and clinicians for work.

Educational policies need to ensure that students in professional schools are required to take courses and have clinical site placements that provide knowledge and skills tailored for long-term care service delivery. The nursing field appears to have taken the lead in this arena. The University of Minnesota's School of Nursing is an example of a professional school that requires all students to take a course that introduces them to the roles, necessary skills, and contributions of nurses in a range of long-term care settings. The course integrates curriculum models with an on-site assignment to a nursing home. As part of the course, students must complete a clinical practicum in a long-term care facility and are assigned to specific residents. Other schools of nursing are beginning to tackle gaps in the preparation and ongoing training of nursing-home nurses as a result of funding from the John A. Hartford Foundation and the Atlantic Philanthropies. The goal is to increase the expertise, authority, and accountability of RNs through the development of a long-term care nurse practice model that promotes the acquisition of geriatric nursing competencies and the special management skills needed in long-term care (Bourbonniere and Strumpf 2008; Beck 2008).

In 2006, the Visiting Nurse Service of New York (VNSNY) and the Hartford Institute for Geriatric Nursing at the New York University College of Nursing began to collaborate on a pilot project to ensure home-care nurses were prepared for geriatrics, with an emphasis on assessment and management of geriatric conditions and syndromes (Flores 2009). The program provides both traditional face-to-face synchronous training and asynchronous Internet training to VNSNY nurses using nationally recognized, best practices training materials.

Both the initial training and the continuing education of direct care workers appear to be inadequate (Menne et al. 2007; Institute of Medicine 2008). There are concerns about inadequate hours and the content of the educational offerings. The Institute of Medicine (2008) recommended that the state and the federal governments increase minimum training standards for all direct-care workers. Federal requirements for minimum training of certified nursing assistants and home-health aides should be raised to at least 120 hours and should include demonstration of competence in the care of older adults as a criterion for certification. States should also establish minimum training requirements for home-care aides.

The Affordable Care Act specifically addresses the inadequacy of training and education of the long-term care workforce by authorizing three years of funding for new training opportunities for direct-care workers. The act also authorizes funds for geriatric education centers for training in geriatrics, chronic care management, and long-term care for faculty in health profession schools and for family caregivers. Another provision expands geriatric-care awards to advanced practice nurses, clinical social workers, pharmacists, and psychologists and establishes traineeships for individuals preparing for advanced degrees in geriatric nursing, including those interested in long-term care.

Make Jobs More Competitive

Federal, state, and local policymakers should make long-term care and direct-care jobs competitive in the health care market as well as with other sectors. Potential approaches include raising wages for long-term care workers so that they are at least in line with their peers in hospitals. Communities can also raise wages for direct-care workers by passing living wage ordinances.

Some states have used Medicaid "wage pass-through" strategies, in which states allocate extra funds to nursing homes or home-health agencies with the proviso that they will use these dollars to increase the wages of the direct-care workforce (Institute of Medicine 2008). This approach has had limited success, has been difficult to enforce, and is not likely to be considered when states are experiencing significant budgetary problems. Given the major role that Medicaid plays in paying for long-term care, such a strategy needs to be improved and reconsidered in the future.

Long-term care staff—particularly direct-care workers—must have access to affordable health insurance coverage. Currently, more than one in four—26 percent—of all direct-care workers are uninsured. Twenty-two percent of those working in nursing homes and a third of those employed in home and community-based settings lack coverage (PHI 2010). The Affordable Care Act could improve coverage for many direct-care workers, but the implementation will take time, and the outcomes are uncertain. Policymakers also need to explore mechanisms through Medicare and Medicaid to increase compensation for medical directors and directors of nursing, who assume federally mandated responsibilities in nursing homes and home-health agencies.

Another approach is to institute payment reform that ties Medicaid rate increases to the success of long-term care employers who demonstrate a significant reduction in turnover, increased staff retention, and better quality outcomes through workplace redesign and continuous quality improvement (Stone and Harahan 2010). Several state Medicaid agencies (Colorado, Georgia, Iowa, Kansas, Oklahoma, Utah, and Vermont) have begun including select workforce measures in their pay-for-performance schemes for nursing homes (Bryant, Stone, and Barbarotta 2009; Konetzka and Werner 2010), but there has been no evaluation of the effectiveness or consequences of these programs.

Implications for the Future

After 20 years of debate about how to reform long-term care, the development of its workforce is finally beginning to receive attention from policymakers, providers, consumers, researchers, and professional and worker associations. Several trends underscore the immediacy of this issue and the need to address the workforce challenge soon. The oft-cited aging of the baby boomers ensures that there will be an increased demand for a trained, competent workforce to deliver and manage the services. The CLASS program, described in chapter 4, may further increase the demand for home- and personal-care workers by providing resources to purchase care in the private market.

As demand is increasing, the labor pool that has historically provided caregiving services to the long-term care population is shrinking. Baby boomers had a smaller than average number of children than their parents, raising uncertainties about the future availability of family caregivers to provide unpaid services. The native-born population age 25 to 44, from which both paid and informal long-term care providers largely come, is not projected to increase over the next decade, and the availability of immigrants to fill this gap is uncertain in light of a lack of a defined national immigration policy. In addition, aging nurses are retiring, and there is a serious shortage of young nurses to replace them. Those entering the field, furthermore, are much more likely to be employed in the acute-care sector than to seek a job in long-term care. As a consequence, long-term care employers cannot rely on traditional sources of labor.

Assistive technologies, such as canes and walkers, and housing adaptations, such as ramps, wheelchair-accessible showers and toilets, and grab bars, help disabled older adults reduce or even eliminate the need for human assistance in carrying out routine activities. Other technologies, such as sensors that help prevent falls or medication reminders that help older adults comply with their medication regimens, may also reduce the need for hands-on or even supervisory assistance (Alwan and Nobel 2008; Center for Technology and Aging 2009). Telehealth and remote monitoring strategies, particularly in rural areas, could create the efficiencies to reduce the demand for human labor. The use of electronic health records that link settings within the long-term care continuum with other parts of the health care sector would increase efficiency among those caring for elderly Americans, potentially increase productivity, and afford staff the opportunity to engage in better diagnostic and hands-on care (Kramer et al. 2009).

Questions remain, however, about the future role of technology in helping the workforce (both informal and formal) to achieve its dual objectives of improving quality of care and quality of life for elderly long-term care consumers (Alwan and Nobel 2008). One major challenge is a lack of awareness among elderly individuals, their families, and providers about the range of technologies currently or potentially available to complement or even replace human assistance. Related barriers are the negative experiences with and misconceptions about technology among elderly Americans and direct-care workers—two populations likely to interact with these mechanisms. In addition, usability challenges, including the lack of adequate technology training and support, limit the adoption of these approaches. There is, furthermore, a lack of consensus regarding the value of technology in supporting "aging in place" across the long-term care continuum of services and settings. The absence of financial and other incentives to encourage investment in the development and implementation of various technologies has also been a major barrier. Finally, critical gaps in connectivity and interoperability among current technologies and information systems have hindered development and implementation.

The Affordable Care Act includes several incentives for developing technology in long-term care (CAST 2010). Provisions include a four-year electronic health record (EHR) grant program to help nursing homes offset the costs of purchasing, leasing, developing, and implementing EHRs; a demonstration program to examine best practices in nursing-home use of health information technology; a specific focus on the use of telehealth and remote monitoring in several home-based care demonstrations; and the expansion of Medicaid waivers to allow the use of these funds to purchase back-up systems and electronic devices to substitute for human assistance.

In conclusion, the development of this workforce needs to be viewed as an opportunity as well as a challenge. The long-term care sector—and home care in particular—is one of the fastest growing occupational areas in the country today (BLS 2010). So policymakers, providers, educators, and consumers must recognize the pivotal role that investment in this workforce can play in driving economic development as well as achieving better quality of care and quality of life for those receiving services. To achieve this goal, the perception of working in long-term care as an undervalued occupation needs to shift, and, at the same time, targeted efforts must be made to address the barriers to increasing and stabilizing the supply across all levels of the workforce.

6

Models of Service Delivery in Long-Term Care

Policymakers, providers, consumers, and researchers have been striving for over a quarter-century to design a system of services that is responsive to the needs of elderly clients and their families and that addresses the twin goals of quality of care and quality of life. Four key issues being addressed include

- how to better integrate acute, primary, chronic, and long-term care services for chronically disabled elderly people;
- how to balance state long-term care systems toward more home and community-based services;
- how to develop consumer-directed delivery systems for most consumers (and their families) who want more choice in how they use their resources and in who provides the care; and
- how to create resident-centered care in nursing homes.

Integrating Acute, Primary, Chronic, and Long-Term Care

As noted in the first chapter, people who need long-term care tend to have multiple chronic conditions and often require primary care and acute care when they are sick (Avalere Health 2008). Financing for acute care is largely a responsibility of Medicare and the federal government, whereas Medicaid and state governments dominate long-term care. This fragmented financing has created silos of care that contribute to the lack of coordination and integration at the delivery level. Many believe that the lack of coordination in service delivery contributes to higher costs and poorer health and functional outcomes. The high rate of unplanned rehospitalizations often is offered as evidence of the failure to coordinate care across the acute and long-term care sectors (Jencks, Williams, and Coleman 2009). In the absence of coordinated care management by professionals, such responsibilities typically fall on family and other informal caregivers who are not equipped to deal with the complexity of multiple service needs (Levine et al. 2010).

Several initiatives at the federal, state, and provider levels seek to manage acute, primary, chronic, and long-term care by integrating services in various ways. The goals for most of these programs are to improve continuity of care and to make more efficient use of existing resources by minimizing use of services in more expensive settings, primarily hospitals and nursing homes. While there is no consensus on the definition of "integration," key elements typically include

- broad and flexible benefits;
- far-reaching delivery systems that include community-based long-term care and care management;
- adoption of mechanisms that integrate care (e.g., care planning protocols, interdisciplinary care teams, integrated information systems);
- overarching quality-control systems with a single point of accountability; and
- flexible funding streams with incentives to integrate dollars and minimize cost shifting.

Despite the rhetoric of integration, there has been a dearth of experimentation and successful innovation over the past 25 years. Barriers to successful integration include fragmentation of funding sources (particularly Medicare and Medicaid), inadequate risk adjustment methodologies to ensure that payments will cover the costs of the most chronically disabled, and the lack of knowledge, information, and training that health and long-term care practitioners need to offer, coordinate, and manage an array of services (Stone 2006a; Grabowski 2006; Grabowski and Bramson 2008). The following section provides examples of programs that have been developed to foster better integration of services across the health and long-term care sectors.

Federal Initiatives

Program of All Inclusive Care for the Elderly (PACE). Perhaps the most well-known program designed to integrate the full range of medical, long-term care and other supportive services for very disabled older adults is PACE. The PACE model is centered on the belief that it is better for seniors with chronic care needs and their families to be served in the community whenever possible. PACE serves individuals who are age 55 or older, certified by their state to need nursing home care, are able to live safely in the community at the time of enrollment, and live in a PACE service area. Most enrollees are low-income, chronically disabled elderly Medicare and Medicaid beneficiaries—"dual eligibles." Through an intensive care management approach conducted by interdisciplinary health and long-term care teams, PACE strives to keep individuals in community care and out of nursing homes and hospitals. Providers receive a combined Medicare/Medicaid capitation payment per client and rely on the adult day care setting as the focal point for service coordination. PACE first became operational as a federal demonstration in 1983 and as of this writing, there are 76 PACE sites distributed over 31 states (National PACE Association 2010).

A 1998 study of participant outcomes found that PACE enrollees in the short term had lower levels of hospitalization and nursing home use and more ambulatory care visits than the comparison group (Chatterji et al. 1998). They also had a decreased mortality rate in one year. Shortly after enrollment, the PACE participants reported more satisfaction with care and with quality of life, but that effect decreased over time. A more recent study compared PACE enrollees with home and community-based care users in eight states and found that PACE participants were more likely to have advance directives and living wills, more likely to receive preventive care, and had fewer hospitalizations (Beauchamp et al. 2008). The study found no effects on health status or satisfaction. A companion study that examined program costs (Foster, Schmitz, and Kemper 2007) found no differences in Medicare costs between the PACE enrollees and the home and community-based care users, but higher Medicaid costs for those enrolled in PACE.

Despite the lack of strong evidence that PACE produces significantly better health and functional outcomes or saves public dollars, the program has received much recognition and congressional support over the years, including achieving permanent provider status in the Medicare program in 1997. At the same time, the program has not grown substantially as is evidenced by the small number of programs operational since the demonstration began over 25 years ago. Some barriers to the development of PACE include the start-up costs and that organizations must assume full financial risk for frail, medically complex individuals. In addition, participants who enroll in the program must give up their primary care physicians, which many are loath to do. Participating organizations must also go through many bureaucratic hoops at the federal and state levels, and there is no flexibility in how the program can be designed.

EverCare. Using Medicare and Medicaid waivers, the EverCare program—developed by United Healthcare in 1986—is a model of integrated primary and long-term care in nursing homes. The program enrolls nursing-home residents in a risk-based HMO, with the nursing home costs covered by Medicaid or private insurance. Teams of geriatric physicians and nurse practitioners provide intensive primary-care services to the residents and coordinate this care with the long-term care services the facility's nursing staff provides. Because EverCare pays for residents' medical services, there is no incentive for the nursing home provider to shift costs to Medicare by hospitalizing a resident.

A team of researchers who conducted a control study of the EverCare program reported that this model, with its heavy use of nurse practitioners, can provide more efficient nursing home care of at least comparable quality to the care nursing homes not contracting with EverCare can provide (Kane et al. 2004). Specifically, the researchers found that the hazard rates of mortality were significantly lower for EverCare residents than for controls. EverCare residents also had fewer preventable hospitalizations, although nursing home quality indicators and functional change were equivalent.

The Home-Based Primary Care Program (HBPC). This U.S. Department of Veterans Affairs (DVA) program provides care through a multidisciplinary team in the individual's home after discharge from a hospital or nursing home (Beales and Edes 2009). The program screens patients to identify those at highest risk and targets care to them, designates a care manager within the multidisciplinary team, provides 24-hour contact, requires prior approval for hospitalizations, and involves the team in any hospital admission planning. Services include management and administration of medication; wound, pain, and medical management; laboratory draws; telehome care; and care coordination between DVA and community-based long-term care providers.

State Initiatives

States have also experimented with integrating services for their chronically disabled elderly populations. Arizona's long-term care system is part of a mandatory Medicaid managed-care program begun in the late 1980s. Medicaid acute, long-term, and behavioral health services are included in the package, but Medicare funding is not integrated. The program implicitly achieves some integration at the contractor level because Medicare services are usually delivered through the organization that provides the capitated long-term care services (Stone 2006b; Grabowski 2006).

Minnesota was the first state to receive Medicare and Medicaid waivers to integrate acute and long-term care services for the elderly in seven counties. The Minnesota Senior Health Options (MSHO) program, developed in 1995, offers a package of acute and long-term care services on a voluntary basis; plans pay for community-based care, case management for high-risk patients, up to 180 days of nursing home costs, and financial incentives to minimize nursing home use and to encourage early nursing home discharges (Kane et al. 2003).

Other states (e.g., Massachusetts, Texas, Wisconsin) have established integrated initiatives combining Medicaid home and community-based waiver programs with Medicare through coordination mechanisms (Grabowski and Bramson 2008). Despite the theoretical underpinnings of these models, however, Grabowski's (2006) review of the research literature on these initiatives indicates that the few studies that have been conducted have been weak methodologically and have produced mixed findings. MSHO—the only integrated state program thoroughly studied to date—saw stable quality of care but higher Medicare and Medicaid costs, though this cost rise may be partially attributable to higher than anticipated enrollment (Kane et al. 2003). The managed care program in Arizona—the program with the strongest evidence of producing savings—seems to have achieved this goal through aggressive preadmission screening and systematic efforts to contain spending on home and community-based services (Weissert et al. 1997).

The Affordable Care Act's New Demonstrations

In an effort to pursue the holy grail of integration, the Affordable Care Act includes several payment and health delivery reforms to encourage better care coordination and service integration, delivered more efficiently and at less cost (KFF 2010). The law also creates a new Federal Coordinated Health Care Office within CMS to help improve coordination between Medicare and Medicaid for beneficiaries dually eligible for both programs. A new Center for Medicare and Medicaid Innovation will also test innovative payment and delivery arrangements that can be implemented nationally without additional legislation (Wiener 2010).

Several pilot and demonstration programs will be supported over the next five years. Initiatives include a pilot program to bundle Medicare payments to hospitals, physician groups, and post-acute care providers (skilled nursing facilities and home-health agencies) with the goal of reducing post-acute care rehospitalization rates and improving the quality of care delivered in the community. Another three-year demonstration provides an additional Medicare payment to accountable care organizations—groups of hospitals, physician groups, health plans, skilled nursing facilities, home-health agencies, and other community-based providers—that are successful in achieving better care coordination and care outcomes for elderly people with chronic and long-term care needs. The Medicare Independence at Home Demonstration provides a payment based on a spending target and establishes a risk corridor for interdisciplinary teams of physicians, nurse practitioners, and other providers who deliver home-based primary care and intensive care coordination to chronically disabled older adults not able to get to physician offices and other ambulatory care settings.

The Community Care Transitions Program demonstration will provide transition services to Medicare beneficiaries who are at high risk of rehospitalization or poor transitions from hospital to post-acute care. This program requires the participating organizations to use evidence-based transitional care approaches, such as the Care Transitions Intervention (CTI) program, funded by the Hartford Foundation and located at the University of Colorado. CTI provides individuals and their family caregivers with tools and support to encourage them to participate more actively in their care transitions. Another evidence-based program, the Transitional Care Model (TCM), targets older adults with no cognitive impairment who have two or more risk factors. TCM is delivered by advanced practice nurses—backed up by physicians—who monitor and manage transitions from the hospital to the community. With an average caseload of 18, each nurse helps patients and family caregivers understand and process information, manages health and functional issues to prevent decline, reconciles and manages medication, and advocates for the patient. Home visits are essential as this provides the nurse the opportunity to assess the patient and the home environment as well as to provide timely education and guidance (Naylor 2006). This model has demonstrated reductions in preventable hospitalizations in three randomized clinical trials funded by the National Institute of Nursing Research (http://www.nursing.upenn.edu/centers/hcgne/TransitionalCare.htm).

Balancing the Long-Term Care System

As noted in chapter 2, the publicly financed long-term care system—primarily services funded by Medicaid—is heavily biased in favor of nursing home coverage. At the inception of the Medicaid program in 1965, the only long-term care services Congress mandated were nursing home and home health agency services. Personal care services were added as an option in 1975. States that include the personal care option in their Medicaid state plans can then use Medicaid funds to cover personal care services. Although technically these services must be available to all eligible individuals, states do limit the benefit through the use of medical necessity as a trigger and through utilization controls. In addition, as noted previously, some states have developed their own state-funded home and community-based services programs.

Beginning in the early 1980s, federal and state governments began to experiment with initiatives to serve more people in their homes or home-like settings and to shift more resources toward HCBS to balance Medicaid spending between institutional and HCBS (Reinhard 2010). In 1981, in the first major effort to rebalance the system, Congress gave states a major policy lever—the Medicaid waiver—allowing states to develop HCBS programs as alternatives to institutional care. The U.S. Supreme Court ruling in *Olmstead vs. Lois Curtis* (119 S. Ct. 2176, 1999) required states to provide services to people with disabilities in the "least restrictive setting" and provided additional incentives for states to offer Medicaid beneficiaries more alternatives to institutional care.

Medicaid can be used as an "upstream" strategy when people with long-term care needs receive HCBS to avoid nursing home placement—known as "nursing home diversion." A downstream strategy can also be used to move nursing home residents into the community—known as "nursing home transition."

As of FY 2009, all 50 states and the District of Columbia offered a total of 318 HCBS waivers whereby Medicaid-eligible disabled elderly, younger people with physical disabilities or chronic mental illness, and individuals with intellectual or developmental disabilities (ID/DD) can receive home and community-based services through these waivers if they meet the waiver criteria (including the need for a nursing-home level of care). Some states have also used broader demonstration waivers to reform their LTC systems (e.g., Vermont, Oregon). The personal care option, available in 34 states and Washington, D.C., in FY 2006, is used most extensively in Arkansas, California, New Mexico, New York, and North Carolina.

Since 2001, states have received a range of grants from CMS and the Administration on Aging to help shift the balance from nursing homes to HCBS. These include

- Real Choice Systems Change Grants ($270 million since 2001) to help states expand HCBS options;
- Nursing Facility Transition Grants to help move residents into HCBS settings;
- Money Follows the Person Grants ($1.4 billion over a five-year period) to accelerate nursing home diversion and transition programs; and
- funds to develop Aging and Disability Resource Centers (ADRC) in each state to serve as a single point of entry and one-stop shopping for elderly and younger disabled people receiving long-term care services.

As of February 2008, more than 140 ADRC pilot sites operated in 43 states. States have also set up telephone and web-based systems to provide consumers with easy access to information and assistance and have developed standardized assessment and program eligibility tools. (See Kassner et al. [2008] for more details on these programs.)

The Medicaid waiver process has been loosened to encourage state balancing activities by providing additional options. For example, while an earlier waiver required applicants to be nursing home certifiable to qualify for benefits, the new waiver uses functional, needs-based criteria not necessarily related to the need for a nursing-home level of service. A more recent option gives qualified individuals an approved self-directed service plan and a budget; unlike earlier waivers, there is no three-year renewal requirement and states do not need to demonstrate cost neutrality.

The Money Follows the Person (MFP) demonstration is the largest Medicaid demonstration program to date designed to assist states in making broad changes in their long-term care systems. In 2007, 30 states were awarded $1.4 billion in grants to pay for 12 months of services for people who have spent at least six months in a long-term care institution (Reinhard 2010). The Affordable Care Act reduced the residence criterion to three months, acknowledging that early intervention is essential to help avoid long-term stays that can make transition more difficult. Under this demonstration, MFP states have planned to transition about 34,000 individuals (approximately half age 65 years and older) from institutional settings to community-based care between 2007 and 2013.

States receiving grant funds are eligible to receive a higher percentage of federal matching dollars to help cover the costs for people moving out of institutions and into community settings. To receive the grant money, state programs are required to transition institutionalized people to a qualified residence in the community. The grant program also requires states to continue providing community services beyond the 12-month period for as long as needed while the participating people maintained Medicaid eligibility. The average number of elderly people that the MFP states seek to transition from nursing homes to the community annually is 4,229 people or 0.6 percent of MFP eligibles age 65 and older (Wenzlow and Lipson 2009).

The number of transitions to date is small, particularly for elderly individuals (Reinhard 2010). Progress, furthermore, has been uneven among the states. In half the MFP states, community-level barriers, such as a lack of affordable and accessible housing and rental vouchers, have hindered states' ability to transition as many people as originally planned. Housing shortages are compounded by long waiting lists for public housing, slow rental turnover among older persons in subsidized housing, and a lack of accessible features that help individuals with mobility and functional disabilities maintain their independence. MFP participants in 12 states received one or more types of housing supplements funded by the U.S. Department of Housing and Urban Development. Although HUD made Housing Choice Vouchers available to nonelderly people transitioning from institutions or at risk of institutionalization, this program did nothing to help elderly individuals. In response to this serious service gap, five states established coalitions of housing and human service organizations to identify housing needs and create housing-related initiatives.

As of 2010, 29 states and the District of Columbia have used the MFP-enhanced matching funds to improve their long-term care systems. These efforts include creating 24-hour nurse help lines, offering intensive transitional care management to move nursing home residents to community settings, providing family caregiver education, paying for assistive technology and home modifications, and focusing on ways to coordinate housing with services.

To date, state implementation of these rebalancing efforts has varied. In 2006, only seven states spent 40 percent or more of their Medicaid long-term care dollars for older people (and younger adults with physical disabilities); the state percentage ranged from 5 to more than 50 (Kassner et al. 2008). While in 22 states, the spending increase in Medicaid long-term care from FY 2001 to FY 2006 was greater than the increase in nursing home spending, 27 states and D.C. experienced just the opposite. Much of the waiver spending (73 percent), furthermore, as was noted earlier in this chapter, pays for services for the intellectually disabled/developmentally disabled population.

Published studies of the impact of rebalancing on costs and cost-effectiveness have been limited and the findings mixed (Grabowski 2006). Early studies of home and community-based services found that while nursing home use was slightly reduced, the aggregate long-term care spending increased. This was due to the fact that states increased their home and community-based services spending on people who would not have entered a nursing home in the absence of these services (the moral hazard or "woodwork" effect). More recent studies have been few and methodologically flawed, making it difficult to ascertain whether these efforts have been successful in reducing costs or producing better quality of care or quality of life.

Mollica and colleagues (2009a) have argued that cost savings from HCBS manifest in the long run. Over time, states that invest in HCBS experience slower Medicaid expenditure growth than states with low HCBS spending. Although Medicaid spending generally increases during a transition, states that commit to comprehensive reforms can realize cost savings over time if they increase HCBS and, at the same time, decrease their reliance on nursing homes (Kaye, LaPlante, and Harrington 2009).

The state of Washington, for example, is taking the long view on reforming its long-term care system. It has reduced its Medicaid nursing facility caseload and directed resulting available funds to support HCBS growth, as Mollica, Kassner, and Houser (2009) note. They also cite Vermont's Choice for Care demonstration program as another example of successful rebalancing. Vermont has created an entitlement to HCBS for participants that meet "highest need" criteria. The state uses a global budget that combines institutional and HCBS dollars in one pot. Over three years, spending growth in this program was between half and two-thirds of what the state had projected when the program was designed. The number of beneficiaries served in nursing homes dropped 9 percent under Choices of Care between 2005 and 2009, while the HCBS in-home caseload grew 155 percent.

Regardless of the evidence, people clearly prefer HCBS to institutional care, and policymakers are responding to these preferences. At the same time, successful rebalancing has proved to be very difficult, and the institutional bias of Medicaid still prevails. The nursing home lobby— historically a formidable opponent to shifting dollars in many states— has advocated against the shift in dollars. Several states (e.g., Minnesota, Pennsylvania, and Wisconsin) are working with the nursing homes to develop financial incentives that will help the facilities downsize and allow the providers to be part of the solution rather than the obstacle. The Medicaid spend-down rules for HCBS clients—requiring that individuals can have no more than $2,000 in nonhousing assets to qualify for the program—have been another major hurdle. To rectify this situation, the Affordable Care Act equalizes the spousal protection from impoverishment between those whose spouse enters a nursing home and those who choose to receive Medicaid home and community-based services. Beginning in 2014, the nondisabled spouse of someone receiving HCBS will have the same income and asset protections as those with a spouse in a nursing home. This change may help to expand noninstitutional options.

The Affordable Care Act includes several policy changes and initiatives to encourage state rebalancing efforts (Justice 2010). The federal government will provide financial incentives (up to $3 billion) to states that are interested in expanding their waiver programs and home-health and personal-assistance benefits under their Medicaid state plans. Participating states with less than 25 percent of their FY 2009 Medicaid LTC spending allocated to noninstitutional services will receive a 5 percentage point increase in the Federal Medicaid Assistance Payments (FMAP) from fiscal years 2010 to 2015. All other states in which less than 50 percent of Medicaid LTC spending was for home and community-based services will receive FMAP incentive payments of 2 percentage points.

The Affordable Care Act also provides more flexibility for states through their various waiver programs and creates a Community First Choice Option that enables states to adopt the more generous institutional eligibility criteria of up to 300 percent of the income threshold for Supplemental Security Insurance (SSI) benefits, thereby equalizing access to personal care services and institutional care based on financial criteria.

Even with these additional incentives, the expansion of HCBS is likely to be slowed as states make significant cuts in Medicaid and other sources of long-term care funding. In many states, the economic downturn and worsening state budgets have strained state Medicaid management resources as well as home and community-based service capacity. This combination has reduced the number of people who can be transitioned through MFP, at least in the near future (Reinhard 2010). In 18 states with MFP grants, the economic downturn and decreased budgets have affected all aspects of the MFP program. State agencies in D.C., Georgia, and Pennsylvania have had to make across-the-board budget cuts that have affected the availability of community-based services. In Arkansas, submission of a waiver amendment to add transition and community-based services for MFP participants was suspended due to prohibitions against new spending. In Iowa, concerns about needing to continue providing home and community-based services after participants complete a year of MFP eligibility have made some providers hesitant to serve them. The future of the MFP demonstration and the other HCBS expansion efforts remains uncertain.

Developing a More Consumer-Directed System

"The 1990s may someday be referred to as the period when the health care and long-term care consumer came of age" (Stone 2006b, 33). Catalyzed by younger people with disabilities who strongly oppose institutionalization and demand a range of community-based options controlled by consumers, a trend toward more consumer involvement in home and community-based services has emerged among the elderly and their families. Consumer direction begins with the ability of the individual with long-term care needs to actively choose the care and setting that fits her needs and preferences. This approach emphasizes privacy, autonomy, and the right to negotiate and manage one's own risk.

Consumer direction is synonymous with the way in which private-pay, long-term care users make their decisions since they have the resources to purchase whatever services they want, in any setting they see as appropriate and preferable. The new national voluntary long-term care insurance program—the CLASS program described in chapter 4—will provide cash payments to beneficiaries. Where public dollars are involved, however, there has historically been controversy about how much discretion publicly subsidized, low-income consumers should have in choosing their services and settings and, in particular, the extent to which elderly people needing long-term care prefer or are able to make their own decisions about care. These concerns include the following:

- Many elderly people are more comfortable with decisions made by professionals and prefer to have decisions made for them.
- A large and growing proportion of elderly long-term care users are cognitively impaired and are not competent to make their own decisions about hiring and firing workers and purchasing services and supports.
- Elderly individuals and their families will not use the cash payments for care and supports but for other purposes.
- Quality of care and safety will be jeopardized.
- In addition, some opponents have viewed this approach as a strategy for depressing wages and exploiting workers.

Over the past decade, however, policymakers, researchers, and advocates for the elderly long-term care population have recognized that consumer direction is a viable option for some older adults. Many policymakers see consumer direction as a potential way to save money through more efficient allocation of resources, fewer administrative costs, and more tailored care delivery.

With the exception of a program administered by the U.S. Department of Veterans Affairs and the new CLASS program, consumer-directed approaches to delivering long-term care have evolved at the state level, through the use of Medicaid waivers, state plans with optional personal care benefits, and state-funded programs (Doty, Mahoney, and Sciegaj 2010). CMS recognizes two models of consumer direction. The first—the employer authority model—gives participants the right to hire, fire, schedule, and supervise aides of their own choosing rather than relying on agency-provided caregivers. A newer model—budget authority—allows participants to manage a budget used to employ aides and purchase related services and goods, such as transportation, assistive technologies, and home modifications. As of 2009, 180 Medicaid programs were in operation (Doty et al. 2010). Although an estimated 2.8 million Medicaid beneficiaries of all ages receive HCBS (Ng, Harrington, and O'Malley Watts 2009), there are no reliable national statistics on enrollment in consumer-directed options.

Researchers who have examined the impact of consumer direction relative to the agency-directed models have challenged the assumptions many policymakers make about the appropriateness of consumer direction for elderly long-term care users. One study of California's Medicaid-funded personal care program that relies primarily on independent providers (i.e., clients hire their workers privately, including paying family members) found that clients using the client-directed mode reported greater satisfaction with services, greater feelings of empowerment, and greater perceived quality of life than those who received care through an agency (Doty, Benjamin, Mathias et al. 1999). No significant differences were found in client safety and unmet needs. Workers in both models reported high job satisfaction, and there were no significant differences between the two worker categories on this measure. The independent providers reported better relationships with their clients than did the agency-based workers.

The three-state Cash and Counseling demonstration and evaluation (Arkansas, Florida, and New Jersey), launched between 1998 and 2000, encompassed the first large-scale, consumer-directed program that allowed Medicaid-eligible individuals to manage the budget for their long-term care services and to purchase services. The results of this controlled experiment, published between 2002 and 2005, provided evidence that quality of life and safety are not jeopardized for those receiving consumer-directed rather than agency-directed services. In addition, the higher-than-expected take-up rates by elderly clients counter the concern that there will be no elderly market for this option. The research team did find that the costs for personal assistance services were significantly higher than for traditional agency-based services. Because experimental program participants' individual budgets were based on the expected cost of the services to which each would otherwise have been entitled, this difference was primarily attributable to the lower likelihood that traditional service users would receive authorized services. (See the special issue of *Health Services Research* 42, no. 1 [2007] for more details on the study findings.)

In 2003, CMS awarded Community Integrated Personal Assistance Services and Supports grants to eight states to help them improve the delivery of consumer-directed services (Kassner et al. 2008). In 2004, 12 additional states received grant funds to replicate the Cash and Counseling model. The Deficit Reduction Act of 2005 further expanded the opportunity for self-direction by allowing all states to offer self-directed personal assistance services without having to seek a federal waiver. The 2010 ACA provides additional provisions for consumer-directed options through its rebalancing efforts (see the rebalancing section in this chapter for more details).

As consumer-directed programs expand within the publicly subsidized HCBS sector, states face many challenges (Doty et al. 2010). Since 2008, the national recession has put severe pressure on state budgets and home and community-based services have often been on the chopping block. These adverse budgetary conditions have intensified demands for cost controls in consumer-directed programs, particularly in light of the Cash and Counseling evaluation that showed their higher costs.

In addition, states seeking to implement new consumer-directed service programs—particularly of the budget authority type—must develop a new infrastructure that has the capacity to develop individual budget-setting methodologies and to financially manage the program. This latter function includes helping participants manage their budgets by performing payroll agent and accounting functions and helping enrollees to fulfill their employer responsibilities by filing and paying their share of taxes on behalf of their caregivers. Doty and colleagues (2010) note that state officials have learned the hard way—chiefly through delays in getting programs under way, slower-than-expected growth, and having to suspend new enrollments while making the transition to new providers of financial management services.

The third challenge is continued resistance from key stakeholders. Home care agencies were the first to fight the expansion of consumer direction, fearing competition and loss of business. Many, however, have come to see that they cannot recruit enough workers to meet the demand for services—particularly in rural areas. Some have also referred their "problem clients" to consumer-directed programs that have more flexibility in hiring, scheduling, and firing. The most resistance has come from case managers and service coordinators who play a key role in traditional HCBS waiver programs. States have recognized the importance of getting buy-in from these stakeholders, as those who find consumer direction inappropriate for their clients will discourage participation. Some states, such as Maine and Florida, have retrained their case managers to become counselors to consumer-directed participants, helping the beneficiaries better understand their role as an employer of a personal care aide.

Culture Change: Resident-Centered Care in Nursing Homes

The Nursing Home Reform Act, passed in 1987, established quality standards for nursing homes nationwide that emphasized the importance of resident-centered care, including a good quality of life and the preservation of residents' rights. Over the past two decades, however, resident-centered care by most nursing homes has been limited. In response to this gap, a growing movement, known as the "culture change" movement, and catalyzed by providers in the Pioneer Network, has worked to deinstitutionalize and radically transform the nursing home environment (Weiner and Ronch 2003; Miller et al. 2010). A "culture change" nursing home is defined as an organization that has home and work environments that include the following:

- Care and resident-related activities directed by residents;
- Environment designed as a home;
- Close relationships among residents, family members, staff, and the community;
- Job design that supports and empowers all staff to respond to residents' needs and preferences;
- Management that allows for collaborative and decentralized decisionmaking;
- Systematic processes that are comprehensive, measurement-based, and used for continuous quality improvement (Spector, Limcangeo, and Mukamel 2006; Weiner and Ronch 2003).

A 2007 survey conducted by the Commonwealth Fund found that although familiarity with the concept is becoming commonplace, less than a third of the nursing homes nationwide indicate that they have "completely" or "for the most part" embraced culture change (Doty, Koren, and Sturla 2008). This figure, furthermore, probably overestimates the level of adoption as the survey participants were limited to directors of nursing, many of whom were likely to report more culture change than frontline nursing and other departmental staff. Among the nursing homes that reportedly adopted culture change, allowing residents greater control over their daily lives is the most frequently cited strategy, while staff empowerment and other organizational changes are less common. Very few facilities have changed their physical structure to create a more home-like environment.

Although the Nursing Home Reform legislation provided a framework for culture change, specific activities have emanated from the field rather than from public policy. The Eden Alternative—one of the early Pioneer Network models—emphasizes community by linking the facility to the outside world, including the introduction of plants and animals into the environment and opportunities for interaction with children and others in the surrounding geographic area (Thomas 1994). Many of the newer models involve substantial physical redesign, including transformation of the dining areas and dining experience, the development of small "neighborhoods" or "households" within the nursing home structure and changing staffing patterns to promote continuity of care (e.g., consistent assignment of direct care workers to specific residents).

A recent evolution of this approach is the development of small-house nursing homes, which are one or more self-contained houses for 10 or fewer residents where staffing, service delivery, and physical design are transformed from the traditional, institutionally oriented nursing home model to a real home environment. Within each home, universal workers are trained and empowered to provide person-centered care to a small group of residents who live together, eat together, and receive services tailored to their individual needs and preferences (Rabig et al. 2006). The most well-known of these initiatives is the Green House, first tested in Tupelo, Mississippi, and currently being replicated through a partnership between the Robert Wood Johnson Foundation and NCB Capital Impact. In a study of the initial Green House development in Mississippi, Kane and colleagues (2007) found generally higher satisfaction and quality of life among residents in the small houses than among their peers in the traditional nursing home comparison sites.

Given the large role states play in financing and regulating long-term care, public policy has the potential and the responsibility to make important administrative, regulatory, and legislative changes that will increase opportunities for culture change. A recent case study of seven states (Georgia, Kansas, Massachusetts, Michigan, North Carolina, Oregon, and Vermont) identified state investment strategies (Bryant, Stone, and Barbarotta 2009). The most common approach is the use of civil monetary penalties (CMPs)—fines that CMS can impose on Medicare- and Medicaid-certified nursing facilities found to be noncompliant with federal safety and quality standards—to support new culture change models and training programs. This approach, however, is a year-to-year effort since it depends entirely on the amount of fines collected.

Recognizing the need to change the work environment to support resident-centered culture change, the Massachusetts state legislature supported a five-year culture change initiative in 2002. When the legislative champion was no longer in power and the funding ended, however, there were no efforts to continue the investment. Oregon and Kansas have created special partnerships between state surveyors and providers that include joint training on culture change so surveyors have a better understanding of perceived or real regulatory barriers to the physical and operational changes needed for culture change.

North Carolina created a voluntary accreditation program (NC NOVA) for nursing home and assisted living providers that have demonstrated organizational transformation that supports culture change. The next step in the process was to tie the special accreditation to increased reimbursement. This phase has stalled because of serious concerns about the Medicaid budget, a phenomenon that is repeated in many states where investments in culture change efforts have come to a halt.

Another eight-state study of rebalancing initiatives identified state efforts to encourage culture change in nursing homes (Kane, Preister, and Kane 2008). These include rewriting Arkansas nursing home regulations and awarding state grants to help support the construction of green houses, developing a competitive grant program in Minnesota to encourage nursing home culture change, developing culture-change training modules in Pennsylvania, and involving state survey agency and ombudsmen staff in the New Mexico statewide culture change coalition.

As Wiener and colleagues (2007) note, these innovations are intuitively appealing but are relatively recent and rare. A national survey of 1,417 long-term care specialists (Miller et al. 2010) identified "senior leadership resistance" as the most significant barrier to culture change, followed by cost and regulation. Although there has been much media coverage, with the exception of the outcomes study cited above (Kane, Lum, et al. 2007), these innovations have not been rigorously evaluated or replicated under varying leadership, ownership, and case mix circumstances. One study comparing an Eden facility with a traditional model found no differences in resident survival, cognition, nutritional status, functional status, infection rates, or cost of care over a one-year period (Coleman et al. 2002). Another one-year study comparing one Eden facility and a traditional model found that residents in the Eden home exhibited less boredom and helplessness than their peers in the traditional facility (Bergman-Evans 2004).

Most of the culture change initiatives have been implemented by non-profit nursing home providers, many of which are part of a larger continuing care retirement community with a strong charismatic leader that also has the land and financial resources to invest. In addition, as the population in nursing facilities becomes more disabled and involves higher levels of medical complexity, some medical characteristics of nursing facilities may be more appropriate than they were in the past and may be compromised by these new, primarily social models of care.

7

Ensuring Quality in Long-Term Care

The quality of long-term care delivered to the disabled elderly population has been a concern for many decades. A 2007 Kaiser Family Foundation poll (KFF 2007) reflected the public's sentiment: 86 percent reported being concerned or very concerned about the quality of nursing home care, and 92 percent expressed significant concern about the quality of home care. A survey of 1,147 long-term care specialists—consumer advocates, public officials, provider representatives, policy experts, researchers, and others—found that 60 percent of the respondents ranked "achieving quality" as one of the top three challenges facing long-term care. More than half (53.3 percent) ranked the quality of care provided in the average nursing home as fair or poor, and approximately a quarter ranked the quality of care provided by the average assisted living or home-care agency as fair or poor.

Almost by definition, long-term care is difficult to separate from daily life. Quality assurance and improvement strategies, therefore, must focus on quality of life as well as the clinical quality of care that is the major emphasis in the larger health care sector (Konetzka and Werner 2010). Despite general agreement on the importance of quality of care and quality of life, defining and measuring quality of life has proved to be more challenging than measuring narrower clinical processes and outcomes (Kane et al. 2003).

Serious concerns about inadequate quality in nursing homes go back to the 1960s and have continued into the 21st century (U.S. Senate Special Committee on Aging 1974; Vladeck 1982; IOM 1986, 2001; GAO 2009). The most significant response to nursing home quality problems was passage of the Omnibus Budget Reconciliation Act of 1987 (OBRA 87), which required nursing homes to "attain or maintain the highest practicable physical, mental, and psychosocial well-being of each resident." Standards were developed to achieve this goal, enforcement mechanisms were expanded, and nursing homes were required to fill out a resident assessment instrument for each resident, at entry and other specified times. As a result, the nursing home sector became subject to more governmental regulation than most other industries.

As the private assisted living market grew over the past two decades, periodic scandals and the growing frailty and disability of the elderly residents have led states to establish regulations for this part of the long-term care sector. While some consumer advocates and experts laud this action, others worry it will contribute to creating a new nursing home industry (Stone and Reinhard 2007; Wilson 2007). And despite state regulation, there continues to be evidence of poor quality of care and quality of life in assisted living (Mollica, Sims-Kastelein, and O'Keefe 2007; Golant and Hyde 2008).

Despite the tremendous growth in home health care agencies during the 1990s, there has been comparatively less attention paid to the quality of care provided by home health care agencies (Harrington et al. 1991; Schlenker, Hittle, and Arnold 1995; Jette, Smith, and McDermott 1996). The U.S. General Accounting Office (2002) conducted a multifaceted study of home health agency deficiencies and complaints, finding evidence that the extent of serious care problems may be understated and that situations endangering the health and well-being of home health patients may occur more often than documented. A DHHS Office of the Inspector General report (2008) indicated that 15 percent of home health agencies repeated the same deficiency citation on three consecutive surveys and that CMS oversight of these entities needs improvement.

Almost no attention has been paid to the quality of personal care and other nonskilled home-care services. Mor, Miller, and Clark (2010) point out that the IOM report *Improving the Quality of Long-Term Care* devoted only one page to quality in HCBS, compared with 22 pages of analysis on the quality of nursing home care (IOM 2001).

The next section provides an overview of the strategies employed by the public and private sectors to ensure nursing homes are providing quality care. This is followed by a discussion of efforts to ensure the delivery of quality services and supports in home-care settings. The chapter concludes with a review of the measurement approaches being used to capture quality in long-term care settings.

Ensuring Quality in Nursing Homes

Strategies have been developed to address the quality of care and quality of life in nursing homes. Walsh (2001) identified three approaches to ensuring quality in this setting: command and control, persuasion (market incentives), and voluntary self-regulation. These approaches and the specific strategies designed to ensure better quality within each approach are described in the following section.

Command and Control Strategies

The dominant model of ensuring long-term care quality is one of "command and control," a regulatory process of *survey and certification* where the federal government (and some states) sets standards governing almost every aspect of nursing home care. Through periodic surveys, inspectors employed by the states determine whether a nursing home is in compliance with these standards. If it is not, a wide range of penalties, from fines to facility closure, can be imposed. In addition, nursing homes certified by Medicare, Medicaid, or both are required to be licensed by the state in which they operate, and staff are subject to federal and state training requirements. This type of regulation, more widely practiced in the United States than in other countries, is intended to deter or remove poor performers rather than reward high quality (Walsh 2001; Werner and Konetzka 2010).

Each state also has a federally funded *nursing home ombudsman program* where nursing home (and assisted living and home care) recipients and their families may file complaints and have them investigated (O'Shaughnessy 2009). Ombudsmen complement federal and state efforts to regulate the nursing home industry through inspection and enforcement. This program, authorized by the Older Americans Act and administered by the U.S. Administration on Aging, typically is staffed at the state level by state employees and volunteers. Ombudsmen often work with the problem facilities to ameliorate consumer concerns about quality of care and life. The program, however, has no enforcement capacity.

In FY 2008, slightly more than 1,300 ombudsmen were responsible for working to resolve residents' complaints in 67,000 nursing homes and other residential care facilities. To ensure that ombudsmen are independent and have the freedom to carry out their consumer advocacy role, programs must be separate from agencies that regulate, license, or certify long-term care services and from associations with long-term care facilities. A key ombudsman function is to visit facilities and residents quarterly. Ombudsmen are responsible for reporting concerns about quality and abuse and neglect to a National Ombudsman Reporting System. In FY 2008, ombudsmen investigated about 272,000 complaints (AoA 2008).

Effectiveness of This Approach. Since the passage of OBRA 87, there has been continuing debate how effective the "command and control" strategy has been in ensuring quality (GAO 2003; Walsh 2001; Kapp 2005; Wiener et al. 2007). Neither federal law nor regulation, for example, provides specific guidance as to what constitutes sufficient staffing. Data from the National Nursing Home Survey suggest that the implementation of OBRA 87 was associated with a 25 percent increase in staffing between 1985 and 1995, but staffing has been fairly flat since then, despite the increase in disability levels of nursing home residents (Wiener et al. 2007). Several studies have found a positive association between nurse staffing levels and processes and outcomes in nursing homes (IOM 2001; Harrington et al. 2000; Bostick et al. 2006). Many clinicians, researchers, and consumer advocates have, therefore, called for more specific staffing standards than those instituted by OBRA 87. In the absence of such federal standards, some states have instituted additional staffing requirements (Harrington and Millman 2001).

While declines in the number of nursing home deficiencies have been reported since the implementation of OBRA, it is not clear whether they can be attributed to the impact of federal regulation, changes in the stringency of enforcement, or limitations in the quality of the data used to measure change and improvement. (Walsh 2001; Miller and Mor 2008). Researchers found that OBRA 87 led to an improvement in clinical quality, such as declines in restraint use and decreases in the rates of resident functional decline and hospitalization (Kane, Williams et al.

1993; Mor, Intrator, Fries et al. 1997). Others have expressed concern that such reported outcomes may simply be the result of changes in the definition of the performance indicator (Schnelle, Ouslander, and Cruise 1997).

CMS relies on the states to administer the regulatory process, with CMS regional offices providing oversight functions. Two studies conducted by the Government Accountability Office (2005; 2007a, b) found severe inconsistencies in how states conduct surveys and a tendency to understate serious deficiencies. In addition, state budget problems have caused hiring freezes and resistance to increasing staff in survey agencies. Regulations implementing the enforcement provisions of OBRA 87 did not even take effect until 1995, eight years after the law passed, in large part because of extended negotiations with the nursing home industry.

Despite key steps taken by CMS to improve enforcement, there is substantial evidence of continued inadequacies (GAO 2007a, b). Nursing homes with serious quality problems continue to cycle in and out of compliance, and few facilities receive sanctions or are decertified from the Medicare and Medicaid programs. The 2010 survey of long-term care specialists (Mor, Miller, and Clark 2010) found that between a quarter and two-fifths of all constituency groups felt that the federal government had done well or very well in establishing quality standards. However, less than 5 percent of consumer advocates and only a fifth of providers and public officials felt that the government had done well or very well in enforcing them. Almost no one felt that the government was consistently applying regulations across states. Mor and colleagues were surprised to find that despite the disappointment with the current regulatory regime, about half of the respondents felt more aggressive enforcement against low-quality providers would be effective.

Despite broad recognition of the ombudsman program's potential to assist residents and to complement federal and state regulatory oversight, limited resources restrict its ability to meet its legislative mandates (O'Shaughnessy 2009). The most recent study of ombudsman capacity, conducted by the Office of the Inspector General in 1998, pointed to the value of the program but noted serious concerns about program capacity and funding (OIG 1999). In FY 2008, 23 states and the District of Columbia met the staff-to-bed ratio recommended by the IOM 1995 evaluation of the ombudsman program (Harris-Wehling, Feasley, and Estes 1995). The ratio ranged from one paid FTE staff member per 791 beds in the District of Columbia to one per 6,692 beds in

Oregon. The program, furthermore, is highly dependent on volunteers, and therefore depends on successful recruitment, intensive training, and high retention rates—factors that vary across states.

Over the past several years, lawsuits have become a growing part of the quality arsenal and have raised significant concerns among nursing home operators, insurers, and policymakers. Some analysts believe that nursing home litigation is the result of quality problems found during the government survey process. Others believe it causes more quality problems than it prevents by diverting resources from patient care. The factors driving the growth of nursing home litigation and its relationship to nursing home quality are not well understood (Stevenson and Studdert 2003).

Persuasion or Incentive-Based Strategies

"Persuasion" or incentive-based strategies—less legalistic and punitive—are designed to generate both negative and positive incentives that influence providers to improve their performance. Werner and Tonetzka (2010) refer to these strategies as market-based reforms, differentiating them from regulation, which is primarily a punitive approach to ensuring quality. Examples include private accreditation, public disclosure, and comparisons of quality information (e.g., state-level nursing home and home care report cards, Medicaid's Nursing Home Compare and Five Star program); incentive payment policies; and CMS-funded technical assistance to nursing homes (and home health care agencies) provided by the quality improvement organization in each state.

Accreditation. Unlike hospitals and health plans, private accreditation efforts have been limited in the nursing home sector. Historically, the Joint Commission on the Accreditation of Healthcare Organizations (JCAHO) accredited several thousand nursing homes during the 1980s and 1990s. A congressionally mandated study found that while delegating the inspection process to JCAHO would have been cheaper than the state regulatory process, this accreditation organization would have had to significantly alter its standards to meet those mandated by CMS, and that JCAHO surveyors missed serious deficiencies state regulators and independent reviewers identified (Abt Associates 1999). Today, the JCAHO accredits a little over a thousand nursing homes. The Commission on Accreditation of Rehabilitation Facilities (CARF), an organization that focuses primarily on accrediting rehabilitation providers, also accredits nursing homes that are part of Continuing Care Retirement Communities.

Public Disclosure. A relatively recent approach to improving quality of care is to provide more information to consumers, their families, hospital discharge planners, and other stakeholders about the quality of care delivered by individual providers through some type of report card (Mor 2005; Mukamel et al. 2008). This market-based approach assumes that consumers need objective information about quality outcomes to help them make more judicious decisions about the nursing home or home health agency use. In theory, market competition would force poorer-performing organizations to improve their quality or lose business (Wiener et al. 2007).

Since 1998, CMS has operated the Nursing Home Compare web site, which provides quality-related information about individual nursing homes. A similar web site called Home Health Compare provides periodic comparison of quality data for home health care agencies. Six states—California, Florida, Iowa, Maryland, Ohio, and Virginia—operate web sites that also provide comparative information on nursing homes (Shugarman and Garland 2006).

A study of a representative sample of nursing homes, home health agencies, and hospital discharge planners found that knowledge of publicly reported quality measures was significantly and positively associated with quality improvement activities (Mukamel et al. 2007). Public reporting had only limited associations with hospital discharge planners using quality measures.

Research on consumer responses to quality of care information has been mixed. While Nursing Home Compare, for example, received much publicity and media attention, a focus group study found that few consumers use the Internet to obtain information for an impending nursing home placement, and few study group participants were aware of the CMS web site (Shugarman and Brown 2006). One survey reported that 12 percent of families of nursing home residents recalled using Nursing Home Compare, although whether they used it to compare quality or simply to identify facilities is unclear (Castle 2009). Stevenson (2006) also found that the impact of Nursing Home Compare on occupancy rates for facilities with high and low quality ratings was minimal.

Several factors may contribute to the limited utility of public disclosure efforts like Nursing Home and Home Health Compare. First, the information is focused on narrow clinical outcomes, is rather technical, and is not consumer friendly. These web sites, furthermore, give little information by which to judge quality of life, an important measure for consumers and their families. In an attempt to replicate a simple star system found in *Consumer Reports* or restaurant guides, CMS developed and launched a Five-Star Nursing Home rating system that ranks facilities from five stars for "much above average" to one star for "much below average" in three areas—health inspections, staffing, and quality measures. This new public disclosure approach has caused controversy, with many providers and some researchers expressing serious concerns that the underlying data are problematic and that the methodology is seriously flawed. Just as with the Nursing Home Compare web site, facilities may rate highly on one dimension and poorly on another. This makes it very difficult for the consumer to judge.

Second, several researchers have noted that initiatives relying on consumer use of quality information may increase disparities if the use and understanding of quality information varies by race and socioeconomic status (Konetzka and Werner 2009). Information, particularly web-based, may be more accessible to educated or wealthy consumers (Jewett and Hibbard 1996). Many barriers exist to widespread use of information technology, and these barriers may differentially affect low-income, long-term care consumers and racial and ethnic minorities who may have limited means to access or effectively use such technology to obtain comparative quality information.

Third, many nursing home and home health care decisions are made on an urgent basis, frequently upon discharge from a hospital. Elderly consumers and their families, therefore, may not have the time to do the comparative research. Nursing home and home-care use, furthermore, is typically geographically bound, thus limiting the choice of providers. This is particularly true in rural areas, where there may only be one provider.

Payment Incentives. Medicaid and Medicare long-term care reimbursement policies are important policy levers because federal and state policymakers have significant control over both the level and methodology of payment (Wiener et al. 2007). One approach for linking reimbursement and quality is "pay for performance," a term used for strategies that integrate quality incentives directly into the payment mechanism. In the past decade, some Medicaid agencies (for example, in Colorado,

Georgia, Iowa, Kansas, Ohio, Oklahoma, Utah, and Vermont) have begun implementing pay for performance in nursing homes (Konetzka and Werner 2010). Many of these programs include a wider variety of measures than Nursing Home Compare, including consumer satisfaction, culture change, and clinical outcomes.

There has been little evaluation of the effectiveness and consequences of these programs. At the federal level, CMS is implementing a demonstration in three states on pay for performance, Medicare post-acute care in nursing homes, but there is no comparable effort to date examining the impact of Medicaid payment incentives.

Establishing a successful system involves several challenges. First, it is difficult to establish unambiguous measures of "high" quality. Related unintended consequences include providers "cherry picking" or selecting less ill or disabled patients and residents to inflate scores; "teaching to the test" by focusing only on reported aspects of quality; and producing data that suffer from coding and ascertainment biases because high-quality facilities—usually better at recognizing and coding problems—would appear to be lower quality than those without these skills (Wu et al. 2005).

Second, such a system might reward facilities likely to be doing well financially because they have a high percentage of private pay residents. Third, if the focus is only on improvement, additional funds could be provided to facilities that improve but are still below average. Finally, assessing how generous the incentives must be to overcome tolerance for profitable poor care is difficult (Kane, Arling, et al. 2007). Iowa's program was the target of media and legislative criticism in 2008 as a result of incentive payments being awarded to certain facilities with negative regulatory survey outcomes. Legislative amendments and agency actions imposed interim restrictions, and the program is going through a major revamp this year.

Technical Assistance. For the past decade, CMS has invested millions of dollars in technical assistance provided by state-based quality improvement organizations (QIOs). Through multiyear contracts, QIOs are funded to work with nursing homes and home health agencies in their states to help them improve on select quality indicators related to clinical outcomes and staffing. Since the contracts are performance-based, QIOs have an incentive to help the nursing homes and agencies improve on targeted measures. Over the years, several QIOs have been awarded additional resources to host web sites that provide educational materials and tools related to continuous quality improvement.

While these efforts have raise awareness about the need for ongoing quality improvement, findings concerning the success of these activities in helping providers to achieve better quality outcomes have been equivocal. Rollow and colleagues (2006) compared measurements of quality before and after a QIO implemented a quality improvement intervention in nonrandomly selected nursing homes and home health agencies. Some participating providers volunteered to receive more intense QIO assistance. The findings suggest that organizations that received intensive assistance scored better on quality indicators than those that did not receive such assistance. As Shortell and Peck (2006) have noted, however, interpreting these findings is difficult, given the severe limitations of the study, including the bias introduced by the nonrandom sample selection, voluntary participation, the possible influence of regression to the mean in a before-after study, and the inability to distinguish the effects of QIO assistance from other concurrent quality improvement activities.

Another study specifically looking at QIOs' work with nursing homes suggests that, based on measurable improvements in residents' quality of life, the QIO program is a sound investment of health care dollars (Shih, Dewar, and Hartman 2007). The researchers relied on a unit of measurement commonly used to assess the benefit of medical interventions—the "quality-adjusted life year," or QALY. They estimated that the investment in nursing home quality improvement, largely attributable to the QIOs, breaks down to $2,063 to $7,667 per QALY gained. However, Shih and colleagues estimated the QIOs' contribution to be 75 percent of observed improvements and did not address the sampling and selection bias raised by Shortell and Peck.

An IOM committee report (2006) called for a large-scale evaluation of the QIO program, an evaluation of individual QIO processes, an impact assessment of selected QIO interventions, and an independent evaluation of the program over time. The committee also recommended a stronger focus on technical assistance to providers, improved governance, improved data processing and management, and streamlined, strengthened oversight of the QIOs by CMS.

Some have called for strengthening the nursing home regulatory process by broadening the survey teams to include social workers, pharmacists, and clinical psychologists to add perspectives currently missing during the inspections (Stone, Bryant, and Barbarotta 2009; Koren 2010). Additional recommendations include better training for surveyors in nursing home culture change and encouraging surveyors to work more closely with QIOs that can act as change agents among clusters of poor performing facilities. Kansas and Oregon have developed technical assistance capacity designed to complement their traditional survey and certification processes (Stone et al. 2009). In Kansas, a special division within the state's Department on Aging was created to provide technical assistance to nursing homes interested in achieving better quality through culture change efforts (see a detailed discussion of this issue in chapter 6). The technical assistance focuses on how culture change improvements can be made within the current regulatory framework. Oregon has developed a formal partnership between regulators and providers where teams of surveyors and nursing home operators are trained together on how to effectively implement culture change within the state's regulatory environment.

Voluntary Self-Regulatory Strategies

Providers have also initiated efforts to improve quality. Six years ago, the three national nursing home provider associations developed an initiative called "Quality First." This grass roots activity includes education and training for nursing home operators and staff, with materials distributed via several web sites and at state and national conferences. Nursing homes participating in this effort have Quality First logos, indicating they support this effort.

Several years ago, a stakeholder coalition of nursing home providers, consumers, direct care worker associations, SEIU, nursing organizations, and QIOs was funded by the Commonwealth Fund to create the National Campaign for Advancing Excellence in Nursing Homes (Koren 2010). Run by a voluntary national steering committee, activities are targeted at the state level, where members of the campaign focus on helping nursing homes improve on select quality indicators (e.g., pain, pressure ulcers, restraint use) and staffing measures (e.g., consistent assignment). Advancing Excellence sponsors periodic webinars addressing clinical and management issues and, for the past two years, has hosted a national conference focusing on best practices. Nursing homes who join the campaign agree to work on improving quality in specific areas and to disclose their outcomes in a comparative manner. The coalition has had several press conferences where the steering committee has announced improvements in pressure ulcer rates and reductions in restraint use.

At the individual provider level, many nursing homes (and home health care entities) conduct periodic consumer and staff satisfaction surveys, engage in on-going staff education and training, use best practice guidelines in particular clinical areas (e.g., dementia care, pain management, falls, and pressure ulcer prevention), and implement culture change interventions to improve quality of care and quality of life for their residents and clients.

Quality Assurance in Medicare Home Health

All home health agencies participating in the Medicare program must be compliant with 15 Medicare conditions of participation (CoP) and 69 standards. CMS contracts with state agencies to conduct initial home health agency certification and recertification surveys to determine CoP compliance. Since FY 2006, all home health agencies have been subject to a recertification survey at least every 36 months. The state agencies are also required to conduct timely investigations of reported complaints and to operate a home health hotline for individuals to register complaints against agencies. In addition, state agencies annually survey a 5 percent targeted sample of at-risk home health agencies. Noncompliance with one or more CoP is cause for termination of participation.

One home-health agency condition requires Medicare-certified agencies to report and transmit patient assessment data, within 30 days of completing the assessment, using the Outcomes and Assessment Information Set (OASIS) (see more details on this data collection process below). For each home-health agency, CMS uses a subset of the OASIS data to calculate a score for 41 quality measures. CMS provides scores for 12 of the quality measures for each home-health agency on its Home Health Compare web site. These scores are updated quarterly.

With respect to the effectiveness of the regulatory process, the GAO (2002) report cited in this chapter's introduction concluded that CMS oversight has not safeguarded patients' well-being. The researchers indicated that state survey activities are insufficient to determine whether problems exist. There is likely underreporting of serious care problems; a survey process that gives surveyors vague criteria for surveying branches and identifying CoP-level deficiencies; inconsistencies in the survey process; a complaint process that does not compensate for survey weaknesses; limited use of federal oversight tools to monitor state performance; and a single sanction that is too limited to prevent a cycle of recurring noncompliance for some home-health agencies.

A more recent report (OIG 2008) echoed the GAO findings. The investigators noted that CMS does not currently use all available deficiency histories in its oversight of home-health agencies. They also noted that CMS should implement intermediate sanctions, such as civil money penalties, suspension of all or part of Medicare payments, and appointment of temporary management for cyclically deficient home-health agencies.

With respect to Medicare Home Health Compare, Wiener, Anderson, and Gage(2009) have noted that few studies have examined whether publicly reported quality measures change consumer or provider behavior in this sector or improve the quality of care provided. They also highlight the lack of consumer perspectives on the web site, although CMS began to report consumer views in 2010, using the Home Health Consumer Assessment of Healthcare Providers and Systems (CAHPS) survey.

Home-health leaders and national geriatric experts have established a Framework for Geriatric Home Health Care to articulate cross-cutting principles that guide all care decisions, to identify key practice areas, and to disseminate best practices for implementing change (Flores 2009). The group has identified six priority areas: care coordination, management, and transitions; medications management; physical function; cognitive function; chronic pain management; and advanced illness management. With support from two national foundations, the Visiting Nurse Service of New York (VNSNY) has begun a second phase of this effort called CHAMP (Collaboration for Homecare Advances in Management and Practice). This initiative includes two strategies—the development of a national Community of Practice to support quality improvement efforts and the expansion of CHAMP multimodal courses to train frontline home-care managers to provide "best practice" geriatric home-health care (see http://www.champ-program.org).

Quality Assurance in Home and Community-Based Care

Unlike the multifaceted approaches being used in nursing homes and, to a lesser extent, by Medicare-certified home health agencies, little formal activity has occurred in home and community-based settings.

Quality Assurance in Home Care

Developing standards for and measuring quality of home care is difficult, partly because of the special characteristics of this mode of service
delivery (Wiener, Anderson, and Gage 2009). First, these services run
the gamut from high-tech medical services to nonskilled homemaker
services; one set of standards, therefore, is not appropriate. Second,
home care takes place in geographically dispersed locations, making data
collection difficult and expensive. Third, quality measures have not been
well developed, particularly for the growing population of cognitively
impaired home-care clients. Fourth, states have been reluctant to develop
a formal quality assurance program that replicates the highly regulated
nursing home setting.

The issue of quality assurance is particularly thorny in the emerging area
of consumer-directed services. As noted earlier, the intent of consumer
direction is to allow consumers maximum control over the choice of services and how services will be provided. Many consumer-directed advocates, particularly younger people with physical disabilities, have opposed
the introduction of formal quality standards, arguing that it is up to the
consumer to determine what quality is. They have expressed concerns that
a formal quality assurance system would destroy consumer direction, particularly the ability of individuals to assume and manage their own risk.

Compared with agency-directed care, consumer-directed services
lack the standard quality-assurance structures of required training for
paraprofessionals, supervision by professionals, licensing, and inspections. Most states have tended to rely on complaints and case manager
interactions with clients to identify problems (Tilly and Wiener 2001). A
substantial portion of consumer-directed workers are family members.
Given that as informal providers, families are not subject to any formal
oversight, it is difficult to impose a more rigid standard when family
members are paid. A growing body of research, furthermore, suggests
that consumer-directed services are at least as good if not better than
those provided by agencies (Foster et al. 2003; Schore, Foster, and
Phillips 2007).

Quality Assurance in Residential Care Facilities

As noted in chapter 2, residential care facilities, such as assisted living
facilities, adult foster homes, and board and care homes, are an important and growing component of the long-term care spectrum of services.

The lack of federal regulation has impeded the development of quality assurance efforts in this sector. Given that most residential care facility residents pay privately for their housing and services, the assumption is that market forces will resolve quality problems. As noted previously, the federal, long-term care ombudsman program allows states to investigate complaints in assisted living and other residential care settings, but lack of funding has significantly limited the role of ombudsmen in any setting other than the nursing home (O'Shaughnessay 2009).

Mollica and colleagues (2007), in their last review of state assisted living policy, report an increase in the number of states hosting assisted living web sites to assist consumers and their families in determining which facility is most likely to meet their needs. Thirty-nine states post additional information online for facility owners, administrators, and managers. Forty-two states list all licensed facilities, 16 states post a consumer guide, and 13 states include information from survey reports and complaint investigations.

Unlike nursing homes, most states do not require facilities to report data to establish outcomes for tracking and comparing with other facilities. The information reported in some states from surveys and complaint investigations is often incomplete, and there are questions about validity and reliability. As of 2006, two states—Alabama and Maine—had developed approaches to rate and compare assisted living facilities (Mollica 2006). Alabama implemented a rating system in 2004 based on survey findings. The scoring system arranges deficiencies into three categories: routine deficiencies that have limited potential for harm; systemic or substantial risk deficiencies that have a high potential for harm; and critical deficiencies that result in actual harm and lead to mandatory enforcement.

Maine developed quality indicators using the resident assessment instrument (RAI) built on the nursing home minimum data set (MDS). The RAI collects information about drug interactions for behavioral health medications, pain, presence of unsettled personal relationships, and the resident's involvement in social activities within the facility. The state oversight agency prepares regular reports that present comparisons of facilities on demographic and other variables reported in the RAI (including age, sex, number and type of ADL or IADL impairments, diagnosis, reason for admission, number of medications, and continence). Facilities have used these reports to develop their own quality improvement strategies and to revise staffing.

In the absence of any significant governmental intervention, two voluntary groups—the Assisted Living Quality Coalition and the Assisted Living Workgroup—have elucidated the values and goals that should inform quality measurement and outcomes (Zimmerman, Sloane, and Fletcher 2008). These include the extent to which services are personalized and provided in a safe environment; whether processes of care promote independence, privacy, and choice; the degree of family, friend, and larger community involvement; and the extent to which services are provided as they would be in a private home. Participants in these two stakeholder groups, however, have not been able to reach a consensus on many key quality issues, including whether assisted living should be defined primarily in reference to the degree of privacy afforded or the specific levels of care provided.

In their overview of quality in assisted living, Zimmerman and colleagues (2008) emphasize that measuring quality involves appreciating the complexity of quality assessment in this setting. Any effort must consider many factors, including the diversity of state and local regulations, facility structure and process of service delivery, resident characteristics, and staffing measures. They argue that nursing home measures should be used or adapted to the extent that they are appropriate, warning that many indicators do not reflect the distinctive philosophy, structure, and caregiving processes central to assisted living. They also note that "the consumer's voice be included whenever possible" and that "data collection does not become the tail that wags the dog" (138).

The State of Quality Measurement in Long-Term Care

The development of a strict regulatory approach to overseeing and monitoring nursing homes and Medicare home-health agencies included a strong emphasis on measuring the quality of care in these settings; far less attention has been paid to the development and use of quality measures in the home and community-based services sector.

Nursing Home Quality Measurement

The On-line Survey and Certification Assessment Reporting System (OSCAR) is a computerized national database for long-term care facilities used for maintaining and retrieving survey and certification data for providers and suppliers approved to participate in the Medicare or Medicaid programs (Wunderlich and Kohler 2001). OSCAR provides information on how well a nursing home has met the regulations and includes data on facility and resident characteristics, staffing, survey deficiencies, and complaints. State licensing and certification agencies under contract with CMS collect and update the data on a regular basis. However, there is often a lag between a facility's survey and when the data can be accessed and aggregated for analysis.

OSCAR data have several limitations in addition to the lag time. There is limited and variable auditing of the data by state surveyors to ensure the accuracy of the information on facility and resident characteristics. Staffing data are not audited and independent analyses have indicated significant data inconsistencies (Harrington et al. 1998). Furthermore, the provider aggregates the resident data, before submission to the surveyors, making examination of subsets of residents impossible. Variability within and between the states in adhering to survey "interpretive guidelines" in deficiency citations is also problematic. Finally, the OSCAR system does not include cost data, impeding analysis of the relationship between the cost and quality of nursing home care.

The MDS is a standardized data set that includes 15 domains: cognitive patterns, communication and hearing patterns, vision patterns, physical functioning and structural problems, continence, psychosocial well-being, mood and behavior patterns, activity pursuit patterns, disease diagnoses, health conditions, nutritional status, oral and dental status, skin condition, medication use, and special treatments and procedures (Wunderlich and Kohler 2001). The MDS was created, tested, modified, retested, and then implemented by the end of 1990 in all Medicare- and Medicaid-certified nursing homes in the United States. CMS designed a revised instrument almost immediately after implementing the initial version to account for the rapidly changing mix of people entering nursing homes and to make improvements based on feedback (Wunderlich and Kohler 2001). Version 2.0 was introduced in 1996 in must nursing homes, and since 1998, all nursing homes are required to transmit the MDS information electronically to CMS on a quarterly basis.

The MDS was initially designed primarily for clinical use to assess the functional, cognitive, and affective levels of residents on admission to the nursing home, at least annually thereafter, and on any significant change in status and to develop individualized care plans. These data, however, have been used to develop specific quality indicators that address resident outcomes, helping to move beyond the surveyors' quality focus on structural outcomes. Between 2002 and 2007, the indicators were quite stable with the exception of two measures. There was a significant decline in the use of physical restraints and a dramatic decrease in pain.

Despite this evidence of quality improvement, however, several concerns have been voiced about using MDS data for quality assurance. First, facility staff complete the MDS largely unsupervised by surveyors, and the assessments are rarely checked for accuracy. Second, some nursing homes may do well on some measures and poorly on others, limiting the utility of a single score (Arling et al. 2005). Third, the modest prevalence of several key measured quality problems (e.g., decubitus ulcers) creates difficult statistical issues in determining quality of care. Fourth, risk adjustment is statistically complicated and open to methodological challenge.

In response to these concerns, CMS designed a new version of the MDS (MDS 3.0) to improve the reliability, accuracy, and usefulness of these data; to include the resident in the assessment process; and to use standard protocols applied in other settings.[1] This new tool was implemented in October 2010.

In 2006, CMS also launched the Post-Acute Care Payment Reform Demonstration to develop and test a uniform assessment instrument—the continuity assessment and record evaluation (CARE) tool—designed to collect longitudinal patient information that bridges the continuum of care and is not specific to any one type of provider (Wiener, Anderson, and Gage 2009). The tool currently captures information from home health and institutional providers but potentially can be used in physician and outpatient offices as well.

Home Health Care Quality Measurement

The Outcome and Assessment Information Set (OASIS) is a group of data elements that represent core items of a comprehensive assessment for home health care patients and form the basis for measuring patient outcomes (CMS 2010). The OASIS was designed, tested, and implemented over a 10-year period to monitor and improve home health care. OASIS data encompass sociodemographic, environmental, support system, health status, and functional status attributes of adult patients. Selected attributes of health service utilization are also included. The core data items were refined through several iterations of clinical and empirical research. A workgroup of home health experts later added other items to augment the outcome data set with items deemed essential for patient assessment. The OASIS items have utility for outcome monitoring, clinical assessment, care planning, and other internal, agency-level applications.

Measuring Quality in Home and Community-Based Services

In 2001, CMS collaborated with state agency associations on a new initiative—the National Quality Inventory Project (NQIP)—to obtain baseline information about state quality assurance systems for home and community-based waiver programs. As a first step, the NQIP partners developed the HCBS framework to give all parties with a stake in the quality of services for older persons and individuals with disabilities a common frame of reference for productive dialogue (Smith and Jackson 2004). The framework focused on participant-centered outcomes along seven design dimensions—participant access, participant-centered service planning and delivery, provider capacity and capabilities, participant safeguards, participant rights and responsibilities, participant outcomes and satisfaction, and system performance. The framework also stressed the interplay between program design and quality management (discovery, remediation, continuous improvement) in achieving desired outcomes.

The HCBS quality framework has been widely disseminated among all stakeholder associations and states and has served as a springboard for the increased emphasis on promoting a constructive relationship among states, CMS, and its regional offices that focuses on quality management and improvement. Several states have also been employing the framework to appraise and modify the management systems for their home and community-based services.

The NQIP researchers surveyed state agencies and found that about 60 percent of all waiver programs serving the elderly or younger physically disabled compiled information concerning participant experience or satisfaction with services (Smith and Jackson 2004). Only 27 percent of the waiver programs collected information about family or informal caregiver satisfaction with services. About a third of the waiver programs reported compiling systematic information about participant outcomes; this practice was more widespread among programs serving developmentally disabled than elderly or younger disabled populations. The report recommended that CMS use the survey results to improve the application and ongoing reporting requirements for the home and community-based waiver program.

As a result, CMS has contracted with an outside firm to provide technical assistance to state Medicaid home and community-based waiver programs to help them design and implement quality assurance and improvement efforts. Focused consultations address person-centered planning, risk assessment, planning and prevention, provider monitoring, the role of case management in quality management and improvement, incident management systems, health supports and medication management, integration of program participation feedback into the quality management system, use of data for quality assurance and improvement, and the design and implementation of quality improvement programs.

The Deficit Reduction Act of 2005 mandated that the Agency for Health Care Research and Quality (AHRQ) develop measures for assessing the quality of home and community-based services provided by states under their Medicaid programs. AHRQ, in consultation with stakeholders, was required to

- develop program performance indicators, client function indicators, and measures of client satisfaction;
- use the indicators and measures to assess home and community-based services and their associated outcomes and to assess each state's overall system of providing these services; and
- make publicly available any best practices identified and the results of a comparative analysis of system features for each state (AHRQ 2007).

The legislation appropriated $1 million for this effort through September 2010.

As the initial step in implementing this mandate, AHRQ initiated the Home and Community-Based Services Measure Scan Project with the goal of identifying and evaluating measures and instruments that could be used or adapted for use in assessing the quality of these services (personal assistance, transportation, case management, home health care, homemaker services, home-delivered meals, behavioral supports, rehabilitation and therapy services, respite care, and congregate housing).

A 23-member technical expert panel was assembled to advise the project team. To date, the team has developed a methodology for identifying and obtaining measures and has identified the data elements to be captured.

In summary, over the past 20 years, increased attention has focused on how to measure and report quality outcomes—primarily in the nursing home setting and Medicare home health care—and how to encourage the use of these data in continuous improvement efforts. As the shift away from institutional to home and community-based services through state Medicaid programs has escalated, there has been a new focus on the development of quality measures and quality assurance systems.

Quality measurement, reporting, and improvement in long-term care have been challenging for many reasons. First, in contrast to acute and, to a lesser extent, primary care, long-term care is designed to help individuals remain as functional and independent as possible for as long as possible. The focus is primarily on maintaining status and compensating for functional losses rather than on cure and restoration. The development of measures and indicators in long-term care settings, therefore, is not as clearly defined as efforts to identify and measure quality outcomes in other health care sectors. Second, as noted earlier in this chapter, quality of life is as, if not more, important than quality of care in long-term care settings. The art and science of measuring quality of life is not as developed as comparable work in measuring quality of care. Finally, long-term care organizations—particularly home and community-based services providers—are not as technologically sophisticated as their peers in the hospital and ambulatory care sectors and have not had tools, such as electronic health records, to facilitate quality measurement and ongoing improvement.

Conclusion

This review of quality assurance, improvement, and measurement issues in long-term care has highlighted the multifaceted approaches being employed in the public and private sectors. It has underscored the limitations and challenges of each strategy in achieving the dual goals of quality of care and quality of life. Miller and Mor (2008) have called for "smarter regulation" that involves improving and maximizing the use of data being collected and explicitly rationalizing the regulator's responsibility to review performance and apply sanctions when necessary. They also argue that oversight should resemble more of a consultancy, with regulators sharing information with providers on how to improve quality. The studies have been limited and the evidence is equivocal on the relative value of the various approaches to quality assurance and improvement. In light of this lack of clarity to help guide decisions and the periodic scandals that heighten consumer concerns, policymakers, providers, consumers, and other stakeholders will likely continue to struggle with this balancing act for many years.

Long-Term Care in 2030

The United States is still a relatively young country compared with most of the countries in the developed world. The aging of the baby boom generation, however, will place increasing demands on our currently fragmented system of long-term care but will also provide opportunities for growth and economic development. Three issues loom large over the next 20 years:

- how modes of service delivery might evolve in response to consumer preferences, ability to purchase care, and changes in public policy;
- whether and how a quality, competent, paid workforce will be developed to meet the service demand; and
- how these services can be made affordable for the majority of older adults who are at risk for needing long-term care and for the federal and state governments that currently foot much of the bill.

The Future of Long-Term Care Service Delivery

While the future of long-term care policy remains uncertain, demographic and service delivery trends suggest that the long-term care delivery system will look very different in 2030 from how it looks today. As noted in chapter 1, a much larger proportion of the elderly population will be age 85 and over and likely to need long-term care (although the increase in that proportion does not reach its peak until 2040 to 2050, when all of the baby boomers have attained that age). These elderly individuals will be more highly educated than the current cohort of older adults, which will undoubtedly translate into consumer demand for a wider array of service options. The increased ethnic and cultural diversity among the future elderly population will influence further the types of services that will be required to meet the needs and preferences of diverse elderly and family caregiver subpopulations. Given the fact that baby boomers and, to a greater extent, their children—the future family caregivers—are currently much more facile with technology than their parents and grandparents, information technology and technological devices will likely play a much larger role in the delivery of services and supports in 2030 than they do in today's market.

A Vision for Long-Term Care Service Delivery in 2030

It is not possible to predict how the service system will evolve. As previous chapters describe, many factors at the macro and micro level will influence the nature and scope of service delivery in the future. A change in policy, for example, could significantly affect the way services are delivered, although policy incentives do not guarantee that a new approach will be broadly adopted and implemented. While there has been an increasing public policy emphasis on shifting resources from institutional care to home and community-based options for low-income elderly individuals (through the Medicaid program) and for middle class elderly Americans (through the CLASS voluntary insurance program), 25 years of effort has not produced the shift that might have been expected from the rhetoric on "rebalancing" the system. Similarly, demonstration activities and specific financial incentives have focused on better integration of acute, primary, and long-term care services for many years, with relatively few successes in achieving this goal.

By 2030, assuming that a more responsive and integrated long-term care system will have evolved to replace the current, fragmented "nonsystem" of delivering services, this system would include the following elements:

The Role of Family Caregivers. Family caregivers will probably continue to play the pivotal role in delivering long-term care services. To the

extent, however, that it is financially feasible and preferred, they will augment their hands-on care and oversight through the purchase of home and
community-based services and technology. Non-kin informal caregivers—
including "significant others," neighbors, and friends—may assume more
responsibilities for individuals who lack close relatives or do not live in
close proximity to family members. Technological advances—including
the development of web-based social networks, sensors, and electronic
medication reminders—will support more long-distance caregiving, leading to an expansion of geriatric care managers and brokers to assist in these
efforts. The ability of technology to complement informal caregiving, of
course, is contingent on the mitigation of the barriers to development,
adoption, and wide-scale use identified in chapter 5.

Family caregivers will have access to more formal training than exists
today, provided through an array of community-based organizations and
offered through multiple modalities, including online. Increased demand
for respite services to allow relatives to have a break from caregiving will
encourage the development of more adult day health centers that are
open on weekends and evenings as well as during the five-day work week.
The federal Family and Medical Leave Act, which currently requires
employers of a certain size to grant unpaid leave to family caregivers, may
also follow the lead of such states as California, which requires employers
to make paid leave available to employees with significant caregiver
responsibilities.

The Role of the Nursing Home. The primary role of the nursing home
in 2030 will be to provide post-acute care to medically complex individuals being discharged from the hospital or those who require significant
rehabilitation following such events as a stroke or hip replacement. These
facilities will also provide a venue for the delivery of palliative care to
dying individuals who cannot remain at home or in another residential
setting. Given the preference for individuals to receive services in their
own homes or communities, the more traditional long-term care services
they need over an extended time will be made available in various home
and community-based settings.

Home and Community-Based Services in 2030. By 2030, the
demand for home and community-based options, coupled with continued policy shifts away from institutional care on the part of Medicare and
Medicaid, will have contributed to the development of a more robust

home and community-based service system than exists today. Home-based care will be provided by a combination of in-person and electronic monitoring systems (including electronic health and long-term care records) to help more of the elderly long-term care population receive services in their homes or apartments. In addition, the expansion of universal design features in building construction and modifications will help to create home environments that adapt to the needs of individuals as they age and become more disabled.

Many individuals will be living in NORCs—naturally occurring retirement communities—where at least half of the residents living in the enclave have reached age 60 and have decided to remain in their homes or apartments rather than move to some other living environment (Baldwin and Poor 2009). NORCs may be vertical—existing in apartments or condominium buildings—or horizontal—across streets, blocks, or neighborhoods of single-family homes. Regardless of the configuration, community members will take advantage of the economies of scale and joint purchasing power afforded by living in the NORC to organize a package of social, wellness, health, and long-term care services available the entire community.

For those who can no longer remain in their own homes, some will move in with family caregivers, perhaps into granny flats attached to their children's homes or a mobile pod located in the backyard (as was recently encouraged through a change in zoning laws in Virginia). Those with no family and individuals who either prefer to live alone or who need a higher level of service than relatives or other informal caregivers can provide will need residential alternatives that offer room and board as well as long-term care services ranging from personal care to skilled nursing. These residential alternatives will be designed to mirror the home environment that the elder lived in prior to the move—including small group homes (such as the Green House model described in chapter 6) and apartments with services. Computer-generated social networks will keep even the most disabled older adults connected to family, friends, and others by creating "senior centers without walls" in which individuals can communicate, socialize, and share information.

The Integration of Services.   Relatively few older adults in the United States today have access to an integrated system of care that is person-centered and that brings together the preventative, primary, chronic, acute, and long-term care services most elderly individuals need as they become older and face greater risks of illness and disability. To date, the models and programs identified in chapter 6 have had little penetration beyond small market areas and have not become normative in terms of health and long-term care practice.

Assuming that the ACA payment reforms, demonstration, and pilots described in previous chapters are implemented and sustained, by 2030, integrated systems of care could become the norm rather than the exception—particularly for older adults and younger people with disabilities. The evolution and wide-scale adoption of electronic health and wellness records by multiple delivery settings could further escalate the development of integrated care. While targeted programs, such as PACE and other Medicaid managed-care initiatives (described in detail in chapter 6), have only served a small proportion of high-risk, disabled older adults, the development of broader, more inclusive programs that offer early prevention and risk management for "well elders" as well as chronic care management and long-term care for more disabled older adults has the potential to be more financially viable as the costs are spread across a larger population.

Who Will Care for Us?

To achieve the vision of a community-based, integrated delivery system for 2030, a well-trained, competent, quality workforce is essential. There is widespread consensus that there are insufficient numbers of competent licensed and direct-care staff to manage, supervise, and deliver high-quality care to the elderly (Stone and Harahan 2010). Without decisive action in the public and private sectors to strengthen and expand this workforce, the situation is expected to worsen as the health and long-term care needs of older adults butt up against population aging. Although technological advances can help to mitigate the need for hands-on staff, the development of the kind of delivery system described above will require significant attention to and investment in the future long-term care workforce.

Some characteristics of the long-term care workforce are a given in 2030. Despite attempts to attract males into this sector, long-term care will probably continue to be dominated by women, particularly the direct-care workforce (90 percent female in 2008) (PHI 2010). The direct-care workforce is already ethnically and racially diverse with only 49 percent being white, non-Hispanic in 2008 (PHI 2010). This trend is likely to continue upward over the next 20 years. Although the racial and ethnic composition of the licensed professional staff in 2030 is less clear, there will be a need for a culturally competent staff to work with a diverse direct-care workforce and to ensure good-quality interactions with a primarily white elderly clientele.

Assuming that the types of policy changes and investments identified in chapter 5 are implemented over the next decade, by 2030, the long-term care sector should be attracting individuals into the various occupations across the spectrum of settings. Growth will be greatest in home and community-based care, with many opportunities to manage and provide direct care in residential settings, individual homes, and NORCs. Colleges and universities will address this evolution of home and community-based care in their curricula and will prepare students to work in settings that increasingly rely on technology. Retirees looking for a second career out of financial necessity or a desire to engage in a helping profession will enroll in educational programs to prepare them for employment. Home care options will provide opportunities for flexible hours and job sharing to meet the needs of many older workers who do not want full-time jobs. Families and friends paid to deliver care through consumer-directed programs will be trained alongside other direct-care workers in how to safely and effectively deliver personal care services.

Those choosing to work in nursing homes, assisted living, and other residential care settings will have embraced person-centered care and culture change. Managers and clinicians will come into organizations with the knowledge and competencies to create a living and work environment that places the resident and family at the center of decisionmaking and that empowers frontline staff to play a key role in the self-managed teams that will deliver care. Staff at all levels will receive in-service training on the latest developments in resident-centered care, how to use the latest information technology and devices, and how to engage in continuous quality improvement. All nursing homes will have nurse practitioners who will either serve as medical directors or work with physicians in that role to ensure that the post-acute population with complex medical or rehabilitation needs receive high-quality care and that they return to the community without the risk of rehospitalizations or other problems.

Long-term care staff will also be part of integrated service teams that coordinate services with hospitals, primary care practices, clinics, and other segments of the health care system. Administrators, clinical professionals, and direct-care staff will have the knowledge and competencies to ensure elderly long-term care consumers with acute or chronic medical needs receive their care in the community to the extent possible and that transitions between settings are smooth and do not result in preventable negative outcomes.

The Affordability Question

Prior to the passage of Medicare and Medicaid, a third of the elderly population lived below the federal poverty level. During the following three decades, that percentage decreased precipitously. At the same time, however, the gap between the "haves" and the "have nots" within the older adult group expanded, and the latest recession—which disproportionately affected current and soon-to-be retirees—raises serious concerns about how future cohorts of older adults facing long-term care decisions will be able to pay for services (Bin Wu 2010).

Ironically, those currently at either financial extreme are more likely than middle-income elderly individuals to have access to many service options. Low-income elderly individuals who qualify for Medicaid (either directly or by "spending down" their income and assets to become financially eligible) are entitled to nursing home coverage and—depending on the state in which they reside—may also have access to publicly subsidized home and community-based care. They also may qualify for publicly subsidized senior housing, although the supply of this residential option is limited. Financially secure elderly individuals have the resources to pay privately for home care, and when that no longer is a viable option, to move into an assisted living facility. Individuals who want the security of a continuum of services may sell their homes and buy into a continuing care retirement community that offers independent housing, assisted living, and skilled nursing to its residents (Baldwin and Poor 2009). Others may create their own "villages"—a grassroots, membership-based, non-profit organization that provides support and community to residents who wish to remain in their own homes or apartments as they age. These self-governing and self-supporting entities are financed by a combination of membership fees, fundraising dollars, and in-kind support. Currently there are 48 fully operational "villages" in the country and over 100 communities developing this model, with the first established in 2001 by the Beacon Hill Village in Boston.

For the vast majority of elderly individuals and their families, however, affordability of long-term care is, and will remain, the ultimate concern. There are uncertainties that contribute to this concern and ambiguity about what type of system will be available and accessible in the future. First, recent state Medicaid budget cuts in response to the latest economic recession underscore the fragility of this program as a safety net for modest- and low-income older adults who need services. Home and community-based services—the options elderly individuals and their families most prefer—have been the most vulnerable in bad economic times.

Second, the fact that the private long-term care insurance market has not grown significantly, even among federal employees and retirees to whom a federally sponsored product has been made available (see chapter 4), suggests that this financing mechanism will not solve the affordability dilemma for most baby boomers. The passage of the CLASS Act will provide a new opportunity for employed middle- and upper-income individuals to obtain modest coverage for home and community-based services when it becomes operational in 2014. Assuming that the program achieves a reasonable penetration rate and is able to mitigate adverse selection, this national voluntary insurance program could potentially offer affordable coverage to a segment of the population that would no longer need to depend on Medicaid as a safety net, freeing up dollars for lower-income individuals in need of services. A cash benefit, furthermore, would allow individual consumers to choose how best to spend and even extend their resources to meet their individual needs.

One thorny issue that must be addressed if affordable residential options are to be available in the future is how to cover the housing costs for individuals who can no longer remain in their homes or rental apartments due to financial or health reasons. Currently, low- and more modest-income older adults who have spent down their assets and income to qualify for Medicaid will have their room and board costs covered if they enter a nursing home. Medicaid reimbursement rates for other residential settings, such as assisted living or adult foster care, however, are generally not sufficient to cover the costs of room and board. And for those who do not qualify for Medicaid, there are no financial mechanisms to help defray housing costs. Recognizing that Medicaid assisted living programs have not proven to be an affordable community-based option, a number of states (e.g., Oregon, Pennsylvania) have brought together staff from their Medicaid and state housing agencies to explore how they can more efficiently package their service and congregate housing dollars to create affordable residential care.

Getting to 2030

To achieve the vision of an affordable person- and family-centered delivery system staffed by a quality workforce, policymakers, providers, consumers, and researchers must jointly develop an evidence-based, applied-policy and research agenda that identifies which financing and delivery approaches produce optimal quality of care, quality of life, and cost outcomes for various segments of the long-term care population. This agenda should include the development of and investment in demonstrations and evaluations that help us to understand how to achieve better integration of health and long-term care services; how to recruit, retain, and train professional and direct care staff; how technology can support care delivery and the potential for older adults to maintain their independence in the community; and how services (including housing) can be made affordable.

Special attention should be paid to how these issues are addressed in different ethnic/racial communities and how the development of a quality delivery system and workforce can best be achieved in rural, urban, and suburban areas. In addition, research needs to focus on how long-term care contributes to the economic growth and development of communities, including the creation of jobs and more stable neighborhoods. To avoid redundancy and the "reinventing of wheels," the findings from this action-oriented research—owned by all stakeholders—must then be disseminated widely and translated into policy and practice.

Ultimately, however, it is the voice of the public that will determine, in large part, how long-term care policy and practice will take shape over the next 20 years. This includes how individuals and their families value the elderly, the services they need, and the people who provide the care.

Notes

Chapter 5. Who Provides Care?

1. Home health care aides typically are employed by Medicare- or Medicaid-certified home-health agencies; home-care aides often are less skilled, employed by private home-care agencies, and hired directly by consumers.

2. Personal communication between the authors and Randy Linder, executive director of NABE.

3. Paul Maidment, "America's Best and Worst Paying Jobs," *Forbes,* June 4, 2007.

Chapter 7. Ensuring Quality in Long-Term Care

1. See "MDS 3.0 for Nursing Homes and Swing Bed Providers" at http://www.cms.hhs.gov/NursingHomeQualityInits/25_NHQIMDS30.asp.

References

AAHSA. See American Association of Homes and Services for the Aging.

AARP. 2008. "The Impact of the Financial Crisis on Older Americans." Washington, DC: AARP Public Policy Institute. http://assets.aarp.org/rgcenter/econ/i19_crisis.pdf.

Abt Associates. 1999. "Regulating Quality in U.S. Nursing Homes." *Health Watch* 3:3–5.

ACF. See Administration on Children and Families.

Administration on Aging (AoA). 2008. "National Ombudsman Reporting Data Tables." Washington, DC: Administration on Aging, U.S. Department of Health and Human Services. http://www.aoa.gov/AoARoot/AoA_Programs/Elder_Rights/Ombudsman/National_State_Data/2008/Index.aspx.

———. 2009. "A Profile of Older Americans: 2009." Washington, DC: Administration on Aging, U.S. Department of Health and Human Services.

Administration on Children and Families (ACF). 2010. "Health Profession Opportunity Grants to Serve TANF Recipients and Other Low-Income Individuals." Washington, DC: U.S. Department of Health and Human Services. http://www.acf.hhs.gov/grants/open/foa/view/HHS-2010-acf-ofa-fx-0126/pdf.

Agency for Healthcare Research and Quality. 2007. "Quality of Care Measures for Home and Community-Based Services under Medicaid." Rockville, MD: Agency for Healthcare Research and Quality. http://www.ahrq.gov/research/ltc/hcbs.htm.

AHCA. See American Health Care Association.

Ahlstrom, Alexis, Emily Clements, Ann Tumlinson, and Jeanne Lambrew. 2004. "The Long-Term Care Partnership Program: Issues and Options." Washington, DC: The Brookings Institute and George Washington University. http://www.allhealth.org/briefingmaterials/TheLTCProgram-IssuesandOptions-453.pdf.

Alexcih, Lisa. 2006. "Nursing Home Use by 'Oldest Old' Sharply Declines." Falls Church, VA: Lewin Group. http://www.lewin.com/content/publications/NursingHomeUseTrendsPaperRev.pdf.

Allen, Kathryn G. 2005. "Long-Term Care Financing: Growing Demand and Cost of Ser-vices Are Straining Federal and State Budgets." Testimony delivered before the U.S. House of Representatives, Subcommittee on Health, Committee on Energy and Commerce. GAO-05-564T. Washington, DC: Government Accountability Office.

Alliance for Quality Nursing Home Care. 2009. "Trends in Post-Acute and Long-Term Care." *Care Context*. Washington, DC: Avalere Health LLC.

———. 2010. "Medicaid's Important Role in Supporting High-Quality Care for Nurs-ing Facility Residents." Washington, DC: Avalere Health LLC.

Alwan, Majd, and Jeremy Nobel. 2008. "State of Technology in Aging Services." Wash-ington, DC: AAHSA.

American Association of Homes and Services for the Aging (AAHSA). 2010a. "Affordable Senior Housing: The Case for Developing Effective Linkages with Health-Related and Supportive Services." Washington, DC: American Association of Homes and Services for the Aging. http://www.leadingage.org/article_ifas.aspx?id=11827.

———. 2010b. "Full Summary of Patient Protection and Affordable Care Act." Wash-ington, DC: American Association of Homes and Services for the Aging. http://www.aahsa.org/article.aspx?id=11169.

American Health Care Association (AHCA). 2008. "Report of Findings—2007 AHCA Survey: Nursing Survey, Nursing Staff Vacancy, and Turnover in Nursing Facilities." Washington, DC: AHCA.

———. 2010a. "Report of Findings—2008 AHCA Survey: Nursing Survey, Nursing Staff Vacancy, and Turnover in Nursing Facilities." Washington, DC: AHCA. http://www.ahcancal.org/research_data/staffing/Documents/Retention_Vacancy_Turnover_Survey2008.pdf.

———. 2010b. "Trends in Nursing Facility Characteristics." Washington, DC: AHCA. http://www.ahcancal.org/research_data/trends_statistics/Documents/trends_nursing_facilities_characteristics_Jun2010.pdf.

American Health Insurance Plans. 2007. "Who Buys Long-Term Care Insurance? A 15-Year Study of Buyers and Non-Buyers, 1990–2005." Washington, DC: American Health Insurance Plans. http://www.ahipresearch.org/PDFs/LTC_Buyers_Guide.pdf.

AoA. See Administration on Aging.

Arling, Greg, Robert L. Kane, Teresa Lewis, and Christine Mueller. 2005. "Future Devel-opment of Nursing Home Quality Indicators." *The Gerontologist* 45(2): 147–56.

Avalere Health. 2007. "Long-Term Care in America: An Introduction." Washington, DC: Avalere Health. http://www.avalerehealth.net/research/docs/The_US_Long_Term_Care_System_An_Introduction.pdf.

Bachu, Amara, and Martin O'Connell. 2001. "Fertility of American Women: June 2000." Current Population Reports. Washington, DC: U.S. Bureau of the Census.

Baldwin, Candace, and Susan Poor. 2009. "There's No Place Like Home: Models of Sup-portive Communities for Elders." Oakland: California HealthCare Foundation. http://www.chcf.org/publications/2009/12/theres-no-place-like-home-models-of-supportive-communities-for-elders.

Beales, Julie Leftwich, and Thomas K. Edes. 2009. "Veterans' Affairs Home-Based Primary Care." *Clinics in Geriatric Medicine* 25:149–54.

Beauchamp, Jody, Valerie Cheh, Robert Schmitz, Peter Kemper, and John Hall. 2008. "The Effect of the Program of All-Inclusive Care for the Elderly (PACE) on Quality." Princeton, NJ: Mathematica Policy Research. http://www.cms.gov/reports/downloads/Beauchamp_2008.pdf.

Beck, Cornelia. 2008. "Geriatric Nursing in Nursing Homes: Initial Results from the Nursing Home Collaborative." *Research in Gerontological Nursing* 1(3): 155–56.

Benjamin, Albert Edward, and Ruth Matthias. 2004. "Work-Life Differences and Outcomes for Agency and Consumer-Directed Home-Care Workers." *The Gerontologist* 44(4): 479–88.

Bergman-Evans, B. 2004. "Beyond the Basics: Effects of the Eden Alternative Model on Quality of Life Issues." *Journal of Gerontological Nursing* 30(6): 27–34.

BHP. See Bureau of Health Professions.

Bin Wu, K. 2010. "Income, Poverty, and Health Insurance Coverage of Older Americans 2008." Fact Sheet. Washington, DC: AARP Public Policy Institute. http://assets.aarp.org/rgcenter/ppi/econ-sec/fs196-economic.pdf.

Bishop, Christine E., Dana Beth Weinberg, Walter Leutz, Almas Dossa, Susan G. Pfefferle, and Rebekah M. Zincavage. 2008. "Nursing Assistants' Job Commitment: Effect of Nursing Home Organizational Factors and Impact on Resident Well-Being." *The Gerontologist* 48 (suppl. 1): 36–45.

BLS. See U.S. Department of Labor, Bureau of Labor Statistics.

Bostick, Jane E., Marilyn J. Rantz, Marcia K. Flesner, and C. Jo Riggs. 2006. "Systematic Review of Studies of Staffing and Quality in Nursing Homes." *Journal of the American Medical Directors Association* 7(6): 366–76.

Bourbonniere, Meg, and Neville E. Strumpf. 2008. "Enhancing Geriatric Nursing Competencies for RNs in Nursing Homes." *Research in Gerontological Nursing* 1(3): 171–75.

Bowers, Barbara J., Susan Esmond, and Nora Jacobson. 2003. "Turnover Reinterpreted: CNAs Talk about Why They Leave." *Journal of Gerontological Nursing* 29(3): 36–43.

Brown, Jeffrey R., and Amy Finkelstein. 2008. "The Interaction of Public and Private Insurance: Medicaid and the Long-Term Care Insurance Market." *The American Economic Review* 98(3): 1083–1102.

Brown, Randall S., and Stacy B. Dale. 2007. "The Research Design and Methodological Issues for the Cash and Counseling Evaluation." *Health Services Research* 42:414–45.

Bryant, Natasha, Robyn I. Stone, and Linda Barbarotta. 2009. "State Investments in Culture Change: Case Study of How States Supported Culture Change Initiatives in Nursing Homes." Washington, DC: American Association of Homes and Services for the Aging.

Buerhaus, Peter I., David I. Auerbach, and Douglas O. Staiger. 2009. "The Recent Surge in Nurse Employment: Causes and Implications." *Health Affairs* 28(4): w657–68.

Bureau of Health Professions (BHP). 2006. "The Registered Nurse Population: Findings from the March 2004 National Sample Survey of Registered Nurses." Washington, DC: Health Resources and Services Administration, U.S. Department of Health and Human Services.

Bureau of Labor Statistics. See U.S. Department of Labor, Bureau of Labor Statistics.

Campbell, John Creighton, Naoki Ikegami, and Mary Jo Gibson. 2010. "Lessons from Public Long-Term Care Insurance in Germany and Japan." *Health Affairs* 29(1): 87–95.

CAST. See Center for Aging Services Technology.

Castle, Nicholas G. 2001. "Administrator Turnover and Quality of Care in Nursing Homes." *The Gerontologist* 41(6): 757–67.

———. 2006. "Measuring Staff Turnover in Nursing Homes." *The Gerontologist* 46(2): 210–19.

———. 2009. "The Nursing Home Compare Report Card: Consumers' Use and Understanding." *Journal of Aging and Social Policy* 21(2): 187–208.

Castle, Nicholas G., and John Engberg. 2006. "Organizational Characteristics Associated with Staff Turnover in Nursing Homes." *The Gerontologist* 46(1): 62–73.

Castle, Nicholas G., and Jamie C. Ferguson. 2010. "What Is Nursing Home Quality and How Is It Measured?" *The Gerontologist* 50(4): 426–42.

Castle, Nicholas G., John Engberg, and Aiju Men. 2007. "Nursing Home Staff Turnover: Impact on Nursing Home Compare Quality Measures." *The Gerontologist* 47(5): 650–61.

Center for Aging Services Technology (CAST). 2010. "Provisions Relevant to Aging Services Technologies in the Patient Protection and Affordable Care Act." Washington, DC: AAHSA.

Center for California Health Workforce Studies. 2005. "An Aging U.S. Population and the Health Care Workforce: Factors Affecting the Need for Geriatric Care Personnel." Washington, DC: Bureau of Health Professions, Health Resources and Services Administration, U.S. Department of Health and Human Services.

Center for Technology and Aging. 2009. "Technologies for Optimizing Medication Use in Older Adults." Oakland, CA: Center for Technology and Aging. http://www.techandaging.org/MedOpPositionPaper.pdf.

Centers for Medicare and Medicaid Services (CMS). 2002. "Overview of OASIS." Baltimore, MD: CMS. http://www.cms.gov/OASIS/02_background.asp.

———. 2009. "Nursing Home Data Compendium." Baltimore, MD: CMS. https://www.cms.gov/CertificationandComplianc/Downloads/nursinghomedatacompendium_508.pdf.

Chatterji, Pinka, Nancy R. Burstein, David Kidder, and Alan White. 1998. "Evaluation of the Program of All-Inclusive Care for the Elderly (PACE) Demonstration: The Impact of PACE on Participant Outcomes." Cambridge, MA: Abt Associates.

CMS. See Centers for Medicare and Medicaid Services.

Coleman, Eric A., and Robert A. Berenson. 2004. "Lost in Transition: Challenges and Opportunities for Improving the Quality of Transitional Care." *Annals of Internal Medicine* 140:533–36.

Coleman, Mary Thoesen, Stephen Looney, James O'Brien, Craig Ziegler, Cynthia A. Pastorino, and Carolyn Turner. 2002. "The Eden Alternative: Findings after One Year of Implementation." *Journals of Gerontology Series A—Biological Sciences and Medical Sciences* 57(7): M422–27.

Connell, Cathleen M., Mary R. Janevic, and Mary P. Gallant. 2001. "The Costs of Caring: Impact of Dementia on Family Caregivers." *Journal of Geriatric Psychiatry and Neurology* 14: 179–87.

Crimmins, Eileen M., and Yasuhiko Saito. 2000. "Change in the Prevalence of Diseases among Older Americans, 1984–1994." *Demographic Research* 3(9): 1–20.

Dale, Stacy, Randall Brown, Barbara Phillips, and Barbara Lepidus Carlson. 2005. "How Do Hired Workers Fare under Consumer-Directed Personal Care?" *The Gerontologist* 45(5): 583–92.

Decker, Frederic H., J. Dollard, and K. R. Kraditor. 2001. "Staffing of Nursing Services in Nursing Homes: Present Issues and Prospects for the Future." *Senior Housing & Care Journal* 9(1): 3–26.

Desai, Mayur M., Harold R. Lentzner, and Julie D. Weeks. 2001. "Unmet Need for Personal Assistance with Activities of Daily Living among Older Adults." *The Gerontologist* 41(1): 82–88.

Doty, Michelle M., Mary Jane Koren, and Elizabeth L. Sturla. 2008. "Culture Change in Nursing Homes: How Far Have We Come? Findings from the Commonwealth Fund 2007 National Survey of Nursing Homes." New York: Commonwealth Fund.

Doty, Pamela, Kevin J. Mahoney, and Mark Sciegaj. 2010. "New State Strategies to Meet Long-Term Care Needs." *Health Affairs* 29(1): 49–56.

Doty, Pamela, A. E. Benjamin, Ruth E. Matthias, and Todd M. Franke. 1999. "In-Home Supportive Services to the Elderly and Disabled: A Comparison of Client-Directed and Professional Management Models of Service Delivery." Washington, DC, and Los Angeles: U.S. Department of Health and Human Services and University of California, Los Angeles.

Evercare. 2007. "Evercare Survey of Graduating High School Students Finds Prospective Nurses Lack Interest in Geriatrics despite Growing Senior Population." http://www.businesswire.com/news/google/20070801005845/en/Evercare-Survey-Graduating-High-School-Seniors-Finds.

Federal Interagency Forum on Aging-Related Statistics. 2010. "Older Americans 2010: Key Indicators of Well-Being." Washington, DC: Government Printing Office.

Fennell, Mary L., Zhanlian Feng, Melissa A. Clark, and Vincent Mor. 2010. "Elderly Hispanics More Likely to Reside in Poor-Quality Nursing Homes." *Health Affairs* 29(1): 65–73.

Flores, Deborah M. 2009. "Annette Totten on a Geriatrics Framework for Home Care: A Quality Improvement Approach." *Journal for Healthcare Quality* 31(2): 54–56.

Foote, Bruce E. 2009. "Reverse Mortgages: Background and Issues." Congressional Research Service Report 7-5700. Washington, DC: Congressional Research Service.

Foster, Leslie, Randall Brown, Barbara Phillips, Jennifer Schore, and Barbara L. Carlson. 2003. "Improving the Quality of Medicaid Personal Assistance through Consumer Direction." *Health Affairs* w3:162–75.

Foster, Leslie, Robert Schmitz, and Peter Kemper. 2007. "The Effects of PACE on Medicare and Medicaid Expenditures." Princeton, NJ: Mathematica Policy Research.

Fox-Grage, Wendy, Barbara Coleman, and Marc Freiman. 2006. "Rebalancing: Ensuring Greater Access to Home and Community-Based Services." Washington, DC: AARP. http://www.aarp.org/health/medicare-insurance/info-2006/fs132_hcbs.html.

Freedman, Vicki A., and Linda G. Martin. 1999. "The Role of Education in Explaining and Forecasting Trends in Functional Limitations among Older Americans." *Demography* 36(4): 461–73.

Freedman, Vicki A., Linda G. Martin, and Robert F. Schoeni. 2002. "Recent Trends in Disability and Functioning among Older Adults in the United States: A Systematic Review." *Journal of the American Medical Association* 288(24): 3137–46.

Garrard, Judith, Robert L. Kane, David M. Radosevich, Carol L. Skay, Sharon Arnold, Loyd Kepferle, Susan McDermott, and Joan L. Buchanan. 1990. "Impact of Geriatric Nurse Practitioners on Nursing Home Residents' Functional Status, Satisfaction, and Discharge Outcomes." *Journal of Medical Care* 28(3): 271–83.

Genworth Financial. 2010. "Genworth 2010 Cost of Care Survey: Home Care Providers, Adult Day Health Care Facilities, Assisted Living Facilities, and Nursing Homes." Richmond, VA: Genworth Financial.

Gibler, Karen M. 2003. "Aging Subsidized Housing Residents: A Growing Problem in U.S. Cities." *Journal of Real Estate Research* 25:395–420.

Gibson, Mary Jo, and Ari Houser. 2008. "Valuing the Invaluable: A New Look at the Economic Value of Family Caregiving." Washington, DC: AARP. http://assets.aarp.org/rgcenter/il/inb142_caregiving.pdf.

Gibson, Mary Jo, and Satyendra K. Verma. 2006. "In Brief: Just Getting By—Unmet Need for Personal Assistance Services among Persons 50 or Older with Disabilities." Washington, DC: AARP Public Policy Institute. http://assets.aarp.org/rgcenter/il/2006_25_disability.pdf.

Golant, Stephen M., and Joan Hyde, eds. 2008. *The Assisted Living Residence: A Vision for the Future.* Baltimore, MD: Johns Hopkins University Press.

Gonyea, Judith G. 2009. "Multigenerational Bonds, Family Support, and Baby Boomers: Current Challenges and Future Prospects for Elder Care." In *Boomer Bust: Economic and Political Issues of the Graying Society,* vol. 2, edited by Robert B. Hudson (213–32). Westport, CT: Praeger.

GAO. See U.S. General Accounting Office and U.S. Government Accountability Office.

Grabowski, David C. 2006. "The Cost Effectiveness of Noninstitutional Long-Term Care Services: Review and Synthesis of the Most Recent Evidence." *Medical Care Research and Review* 63(1): 3–28.

Grabowski, David C., and Jeffrey Bramson. 2008. "State Initiatives to Integrate the Medicare and Medicaid Programs for Dually Eligible Beneficiaries." *Generations* 32(3): 54–60.

Haley, Barbara A., Robert W. Gray, Lydia B. Taghavi, Dianne T. Thompson, Deborah Devine, Abdollah H. Haghighi, and Seth R. Marcus. 2008. "Section 202 Supportive Housing for the Elderly: Program Status and Performance Measurement." Washington, DC: U.S. Department of Housing and Urban Development, Office of Policy Development and Research. http://www.huduser.org/portal/publications/hsgspec/sec_202.html/.

Hamilton, Nadine, and Anita S. Tesh. 2002. "The North Carolina EDEN Coalition: Facilitating Environmental Transformation." *Journal of Gerontological Nursing* 28(3): 35–40.

Han, Beth, Al Sirrocco, and Robin Remsburg. 2003. "Developing Typology of Long-Term Care Residential Places: The First Step." Hyattsville, MD: National Center for Health Statistics, Center for Disease Control and Prevention.

Harahan, Mary F., and Robyn I. Stone. 2009. "Who Will Care? Building the Geriatric Long-Term Care Workforce." In *Boomer Bust? Economic and Political Issues of the Graying Society,* vol. 2, edited by Robert B. Hudson (233–53). Westport, CT: Praeger Publishing.

Harahan, Mary F., Alisha Sanders, and Robyn I Stone. 2006. "Linking Affordable Housing with Services: A Long-Term Care Option for Low and Modest Income Seniors." *Seniors Housing and Care Journal* 14(1): 35–46.

Harrington, Charlene, and M. Millman. 2001. "Nursing Home Staffing Standards in State Statutes and Regulations." Menlo Park, CA: Henry J. Kaiser Family Foundation.

Harrington, Charlene, Helen Carrillo, Joe Mullan, and James H. Swan. 1998. "Nursing Facility Staffing in the States: The 1991 to 1995 Period." *Medical Care Research and Review* 55(3): 334–63.

Harrington, Charlene, Leslie A. Grant, Stanley R. Ingman, and Sherry A. Hobson. 1991. "The Regulation of Home Health Care Quality." *Journal of Applied Gerontology* 10:53–70.

Harrington, Charlene, David Zimmerman, Sarita L. Karon, James Robinson, and Patricia Beutel. 2000. "Nursing Home Staffing and Its Relationship to Deficiencies." *The Journals of Gerontology: Series B* 55(5): S278–87.

Harris-Wehling, Jo, Jill C. Feasley, and Carol L. Estes, eds. 1995. *Real People, Real Problems: An Evaluation of the Long-Term Care Ombudsman Programs of the Older Americans Act.* Washington, DC: Institute of Medicine. http://www.nap.edu/catalog.php?record_id=9059.

Hartman, Micah, Anne Martin, Patricia McDonnell, and Aaron Catlin. 2009. "National Health Spending in 2007: Slower Drug Spending Contributes to Lowest Rate of Overall Growth since 1998." *Health Affairs* 28(1): 246–61.

Harvath, Theresa A., Kristen Swafford, Kathryn Smith, Lois L. Miller, Miriam Volpin, Kathryn Sexon, Diana White, and Heather A. Young. 2008. "Enhancing Nursing Leadership in Long-Term Care: A Review of the Literature." *Research in Gerontological Nursing* 1(3).

Hawes, Catherine, Judith B. Wildfire, and Linda J. Lux. 1993. "The Regulation of Board and Care Homes, Results of a 50-State Survey: National Summary." Washington, DC: American Association of Retired Persons.

Hawes, Catherine, Charles D. Phillips, Miriam Rose, Scott Holan, and Michael Sherman. 2003. "A National Survey of Assisted Living Facilities." *The Gerontologist* 43(6): 875–82.

Houser, Ari N. 2007. "Long-Term Care Research Report." Washington, DC: AARP.

Houser, Ari N., and Mary Jo Gibson. 2008. "Valuing the Invaluable: The Economic Value of Family Caregiving." *Insight on the Issues* 13. Washington, DC: AARP.

Houser, Ari N., Wendy Fox-Grage, and Mary Jo Gibson. 2009. *Across the States: Profiles of Long-Term Care and Independent Living,* 8th edition. Washington, DC: AARP Public Policy Institute. http://www.aarp.org/acrossthestates.

Howes, Candace. 2008. "Love, Money, or Flexibility: What Motivates People to Work in Consumer-Directed Home Care?" *The Gerontologist* 48(Special Issue 1): 46–59.

Huskamp, Haiden A., David G. Stevenson, Michael E. Chernew, and Joseph P. Newhouse. 2010. "A New Medicare End of Life Benefit for Nursing Home Residents." *Health Affairs* 29(1): 130–35.

Hwalek, Melanie, Victoria Straub, and Karen Kosniewski. 2008. "Older Workers: An Opportunity to Expand the Long-Term Care/Direct Care Labor Force." *The Gerontologist* 48(Suppl. 1): 90–103.

Institute of Medicine (IOM). 1986. *Improving the Quality of Care in Nursing Homes.* Washington, DC: National Academies Press.

———. 2001. *Improving the Quality of Long-Term Care.* Washington, DC: National Academies Press.

———. 2006. "Medicare's Quality Improvement Organization Program: Maximizing Potential." Washington, DC: National Academies of Science.

———. 2008. *Retooling for an Aging America.* Washington, DC: National Academies Press.

Interagency Forum on Aging Related Statistics. 2010. "Older Americans 2010: Key Indicators of Well-Being." Washington, DC: Government Printing Office.

Intrator, Orna, Zhanlian Feng, Vincent Mor, David Gifford, Meg Bourbonniere, and Jacqueline Zinn. 2005. "The Employment of Nurse Practitioners and Physician Assistants in U.S. Nursing Homes." *The Gerontologist* 45:486–95.

IOM. *See* Institute of Medicine.

Jencks, Stephen F., Mark V. Williams, and Eric A. Coleman. 2009. "Rehospitalizations among Patients in the Medicare Fee-for-Service Program." *New England Journal of Medicine* 360:1418–28.

Jette, Alan M., Kevin W. Smith, and Susan M. McDermott. 1996. "Quality of Medicare-Reimbursed Home Health Care." *The Gerontologist* 36(4): 492–501.

Jewett, Jacquelyn J., and Judith H. Hibbard. 1996. "Comprehension of Quality Care Indicators: Differences among Privately Insured, Publicly Insured, and Uninsured." *Health Care Financing Review* 18(1): 75–94.

Johnson, Richard W., and Joshua M. Wiener. 2006. "A Profile of Frail Older Americans and Their Caregivers." Occasional Paper 8. Washington, DC: The Urban Institute. http://www.urban.org/url.cfm?ID=311284.

Johnson, Richard W., Desmond Toohey, and Joshua M. Wiener. 2007. "Meeting the Long-Term Care Needs of the Baby Boomers: How Changing Families Will Affect Paid Helpers and Institutions." Discussion Paper 07-04. Washington, DC: The Urban Institute. http://www.urban.org/url.cfm?ID=311451.

Justice, Diane. 2010. "Long-Term Services and Supports and Chronic Care Coordination: Policy Advances Enacted by the Patient Protection and Affordable Care Act." Washington, DC: National Academy for State Health Policy.

Kaiser Family Foundation (KFF). 2007. "Kaiser Public Opinion Spotlight: The Public's Views on Long-Term Care." Menlo Park, CA: Kaiser Family Foundation. http://www.kff.org/spotlight/longterm/index.cfm.

———. 2010. "Medicare Spending and Financing." Fact Sheet. Menlo Park, CA: Kaiser Family Foundation. http://www.kff.org/Medicare/upload/7305-05.pdf.

Kane, Robert L., Shannon Flood, Boris Bershadsky, and Gale Keckhafer. 2004. "Effect of an Innovative Medicare Managed Care Program on the Quality of Care for Nursing Home Residents." *The Gerontologist* 44(1): 95–103.

Kane, Robert L., Patricia Homyak, Boris Bershadsky, Yat-Sang Lum, and Mir Said Siadaty. 2003. "Outcomes of Managed Care of Dually Eligible Older Persons." *The Gerontologist* 43(2): 165–74.

Kane, Robert L., Carter C. Williams, T. Franklin Williams, and Rosalie A. Kane. 1993. "Restraining Restraints: Changes in a Standard of Care." *Annual Review of Public Health* 14:545–84.

Kane, Robert L., Greg Arling, Christine Mueller, Robert Held, and Valerie Cooke. 2007. "A Quality-Based Payment Strategy for Nursing Home Care in Minnesota." *The Gerontologist* 47:108–115.

Kane, Rosalie A., Robert L. Kane, and Richard C. Ladd. 1998. *The Heart of Long-Term Care.* London: Oxford University Press.

Kane, Rosalie A., R. Preister, and Robert L. Kane. 2008. "The Future of the Nursing Home in a Rebalanced Long-Term Services and Supports (LTSS) System." Topic Paper No. 5. University of Minnesota. http://www.sph.umn.edu/hpm/ltcresourcecenter/research/rebalancing/attachments/topicpapers/Topic_5_Future_of_the_Nursing_Home_in_a_Rebalanced_System.pdf.

Kane, Rosalie A., Terry Y. Lum, Lois J. Cutler, Howard B. Degenholtz, and Tzy-Chyi Yu. 2007. "Resident Outcomes in Small-House Nursing Homes: A Longitudinal Evaluation of the Initial Green House Program." *Journal of the American Geriatrics Society* 55(6): 832–39.

Kane, Rosalie A., Kristen C. Kling, Boris Bershadsky, Robert L. Kane, Katherine Giles, Howard B. Defenholtz, Jiexin Liu, and Lois J. Cutler. 2003. "Quality of Life Measures for Nursing Home Residents." *Journal of Gerontology* 58(3): 240–48.

Kapp, Marshall B. 2005. "Improving the Quality of Nursing Homes: Introduction to a Symposium on the Role of Regulation." *Journal of Legal Medicine* 26(1): 1–8.

Kasper, Judith, and Molly O'Malley. 2007. "Changes in Characteristics, Needs, and Payment for Care of Elderly Nursing Home Residents: 1999 to 2004." Washington, DC: Kaiser Commission on Medicaid and the Uninsured. http://www.kff.org/medicaid/7663.cfm.

Kassner, Enid, Susan Reinhard, Wendy Fox-Grage, Ari Houser, Barbara Coleman, and Dann Milne. 2008. "A Balancing Act: State Long-Term Care Reform." Washington, DC: AARP.

Kaye, H. Stephen, Charlene Harrington, and Mitchell P. LaPlante. 2010. "Long-Term Care: Who Gets It, Who Provides It, Who Pays, and How Much?" *Health Affairs* 29(1): 11–21.

Kaye, H. Stephen, Mitchell P. LaPlante, and Charlene Harrington. 2009. "Do Noninstitutional Long-Term Care Services Reduce Medicaid Spending?" *Health Affairs* 28(1): 262–72.

Kemper, Peter, Harriet L. Komisar, and Lisa Alexcih. 2005. "Long-Term Care over an Uncertain Future: What Can Current Retirees Expect?" *Inquiry* 42(4): 335–50.

KFF. See Kaiser Family Foundation.

Kochera, Andrew, and Kim Bright. 2006. "Livable Communities for Older People." *Generations* 29(4): 32–36.

Komisar, Harriet L., Ann Tumlinson, Judy Feder, and Shelia Burke. 2009. "Long-Term Care in Health Care Reform: Policy Options to Improve Both." Long Beach, CA: SCAN Foundation. http://www.avalerehealth.net/research/docs/Policy_Brief_with_Cover_FINAL_July_16%202009.pdf.

Konetzka, R. Tamara, and Rachel M. Werner. 2009. "Disparities in Long-Term Care: Building Equity into Market-Based Reforms." *Medical Care Research Review* 66(5): 491–521.

———. 2010. "Applying Market-Based Reforms to Long-Term Care." *Health Affairs* 29(1): 74–80.

Koren, Mary Jane. 2010. "Improving Quality in Long-Term Care." *Medical Care Research and Review* 67(4): 141S–51S.

Kramer, Andrew, Angela A. Richard, Anne Epstein, Dennis Winn, and Karis May. 2009. "Understanding the Costs and Benefits of Health Information Technology in Nursing Homes and Home Health Agencies: Case Study Findings." Washington, DC: U.S. Department of Health and Human Services. http://aspe.hhs.gov/daltcp/reports/2009/HITcsf.pdf.

Lakdawalla, Darius, and Tomas Philipson. 2002. "The Rise in Old-Age Longevity and the Market for Long-Term Care." *American Economic Review* 92(1): 295–306.

Lakdawalla, Darius, Jayanta Bhattacharya, and Dana P. Goldman. 2004. "Are the Young Becoming More Disabled?" *Health Affairs* 23(1): 168–76.

Leutz, Walter N. 2007. "Immigration and the Elderly: Foreign-Born Workers in Long-Term Care." *Immigration Policy in Focus* 5(12). Washington, DC: American Immigration Law Foundation. http://www.immigrationpolicy.org/special-reports/immigration-and-elderly-foreign-born-workers-long-term-care.

Levenson, Steven A., and Dana A. Saffel. 2007. "The Consultant Pharmacist and the Physician in the Nursing Home: Roles, Relationships, and a Recipe for Success." *The Consultant Pharmacist* 22(1): 71–82.

Levine, Carol, Deborah Halper, Ariella Peist, and David A. Gould. 2010. "Bridging Troubled Waters: Family Caregivers, Transitions, and Long-Term Care." *Health Affairs* 29(1): 116–24.

Levy, Cari, Anne Epstein, Lori-Ann Landry, Andrea Kramer, Jennie Harvell, and Charlene Liggings. 2005. "Literature Review and Synthesis of Physician Practices in Nursing Homes." Washington, DC: U.S. Department of Health and Human Services.

The Lewin Group. 2010. "Medicaid and Long-Term Care: New Challenges, New Opportunities." Falls Church, VA: The Lewin Group.

LifePlans. 2007. "Who Buys Long-Term Care Insurance? A 15-Year Study of Buyers and Non-Buyers, 1990–2005." Washington, DC: America's Health Insurance Plans. http://www.ahipresearch.org/pdfs/LTC_Buyers_Guide.pdf.

Lindner, Randy L. 2007. Testimony of Randy L. Lindner, Executive Director, National Association of Boards of Examiners of Long Term Care Administrators. http://www.qualitylongtermcarecommission.org/pdf/randy_lindner_testimony.pdf.

Lo Sasso, Anthony T., and Richard W. Johnson. 2002. "Does Informal Care from Adult Children Reduce Nursing Home Admissions for the Elderly?" *Inquiry* 39(3): 279–97.

Manton, Kenneth G., XiLiang Gu, and Vicki L. Lamb. 2006. "Change in Chronic Disability from 1982 to 2004–2005 as Measured by Long-Term Changes in Function and Health in the U.S. Elderly Population." *Proceedings of the National Academy of Sciences* 103(48): 18374–79.

Martin, Susan F., B. Lindsey Lowell, Elzbieta M. Gozdiak, Micah Bump, and Mary E. Breeding. 2009. "The Role of Migrant Care Workers in Aging Societies: Report on Research Findings in the United States." Washington, DC: Institute for the Study of International Migration, Georgetown University. http://isim.georgetown.edu/Publications/GrantReports/ElderCareReport.pdf.

McNichol, Elizabeth, Phil Oliff, and Nicholas Johnson. 2010. "Recession Continues to Batter State Budgets; State Responses Could Slow Recovery." Center on Budget and Policy Priorities. http://www.cbpp.org/cms/?fa17=view&id=711.

Menne, Heather L., Farida K. Ejaz, Linda S. Noelker, and James A. Jones. 2007. "Direct Care Workers' Recommendations for Training and Continuing Education." *Gerontology and Geriatrics Education* 28(2): 91–108.

Meier, Dianne E., Betty Lim, and Melissa D. Carlson. 2010. "Raising the Standard: Palliative Care in Nursing Homes." *Health Affairs* 29(1): 136–40.

Metlife Mature Market Institute. 2008. "National Survey of Nursing Home and Assisted Living Costs." http://www.metlife.com/assets/cao/mmi/publications/mmi-pressroom/mmi-press-releases-2008-nhal-costs.pdf.

Miller, Edward Alan, and Vincent Mor. 2008. "Balancing Regulatory Controls and Incentives: Toward Smarter and More Transparent Oversight in Long-Term Care." *Journal of Politics, Policy and Law* 33(2): 249–79.

Miller, Susan C., Edward Alan Miller, Hye-Young Jung, Samantha Sterns, Melissa A. Clark, and Vincent Mor. 2010. "Nursing Home Organizational Change: The 'Culture Change' Movement as Viewed by Long-Term Care Specialists." *Medical Care Research and Review* 67(4 Suppl.): 65S–81S.

Mitchell, Susan L., Joan M. Teno, Dan K. Kiely, Michele L. Shaffer, Richard N. Jones, Holly G. Prigerson, Ladislav Volicer, Jane L. Givens, and Mary Beth Hamel. 2009. "The Clinical Course of Advanced Dementia." *New England Journal of Medicine* 361(16): 1529–38.

Mollica, Robert L. 2006. "Residential Care and Assisted Living: State Oversight Practices and State Information Available to Consumers." Rockville, MD: Agency for Healthcare Research and Quality.

Mollica, Robert L., Maureen Booth, Carolyn Gray, and Kristin Sims-Kastelein. 2008. "Adult Foster Care: A Resource for Older Adults." New Brunswick, NJ: Rutgers Center for State Healthy Policy.

Mollica, Robert L., Kristin Sims-Kastelein, and Janet O'Keefe. 2007. "Residential Care and Assisted Living Compendium: 2007." Washington, DC: U.S. Department of Health and Human Services.

Mollica, Robert L., Kristin Sims-Kastelein, and Enid Kassner. 2009. "State-Funded Home and Community-Based Services Programs for Older Adults." Washington, DC: AARP Public Policy Institute. http://share.aarp.org/research/ppi/ltc/hcbs/articles/2009_06_hcbs.html.

Mollica, Robert L., Kristin Sims-Kastelein, Michael Cheek, Candice Baldwin, Jennifer Farnham, Susan Reinhard, and Jean Accius. 2009. "Building Adult Foster Care: What States Can Do." Washington, DC: AARP Public Policy Institute. http://www.aarp.org/ppi.

Mollica, Robert L., Enid Kassner, Lina Walker, and Ari Houser. 2009. "Taking the Long View: Investing in Medicaid Home and Community-Based Services Is Cost Effective." *Insight on the Issues* 126. Washington, DC: AARP Public Policy Institute. http://assets.aarp.org/rgcenter/il/i26_hcbs.pdf.

Montgomery, Rhonda J.V., Lyn Holley, Jerome Deichert, and Karl Kosloski. 2005. "A Profile of Home Care Workers from the 2000 Census: How It Changes What We Know." *The Gerontologist* 45(5): 593–600.

Moore, J., and L. Payne. 2002. "State Responses to Health Worker Shortages: Results of the 2002 Survey of States." Rensselaer, NY: Center for Health Workforce Studies, School of Public Health, SUNY Albany.

Mor, Vincent. 2005. "Improving the Quality of Long-Term Care with Better Information." *The Milbank Quarterly* 83(3): 333–64.

Mor, Vincent, Edward Alan Miller, and Melissa Clark. 2010. "The Taste for Regulation in Long-Term Care." *Medical Care Research Review* 67:38S–64S.

Mor, Vincent, Orna Intrator, Brant E. Fries, C. Phillips, Joan M. Teno, J. Hiris, C. Hawes, and J. Morris. 1997. "Changes in Hospitalization Associated with Introducing the Resident Assessment Instrument." *Journal of the American Geriatrics Society* 45(8): 1002–1010.

Mukamel, Dana B., William D. Spector, Jacqueline S. Zinn, Lynn Huang, David L. Weimer, and Ann Dozier. 2007. "Nursing Homes' Response to the Nursing Home Compare Report Card." *Journal of Gerontology* 62(4): S218–25.

Mukamel, Dana B., David L. Wiemer, William D. Spector, Heather Ladd, and Jacqueline S. Zinn. 2008. "Publication of Quality Report Cards and Trends in Reported Quality Measures in Nursing Homes." *Health Services Research* 43(4): 1244–62.

Murtaugh, Christopher, Timothy Peng, Annette Totten, Beth Costello, Stanley Moore, and Hakan Aykan. 2009. "Complexity in Geriatric Home Healthcare." *Journal for Healthcare Quality* 31(2): 34–43.

NASUA. See National Association of State Units on Aging.

NASW. See National Association of Social Workers.

National Academy on an Aging Society. 2010. "Bringing CLASS to Long-Term Care through the Affordable Care Act." *Public Policy and Aging Report* 20(2). Washington, DC: National Academy on an Aging Society.

National Association of Home Care and Hospice. 2009. "Basic Statistics about Home Care: Updated 2010." Washington, DC: National Association of Home Care and Hospice. http://www.nahc.org/facts/10HC_Stats.pdf.

National Association of Social Workers (NASW). 2006. "Assuring the Sufficiency of a Frontline Workforce: A National Study of Licensed Social Workers—Special Report: Social Work Services for Older Adults." Washington, DC: National Association of Social Workers, Center for Workforce Studies. http://workforce.socialworkers.org/studies/aging/aging.pdf.

National Association of State Units on Aging (NASUA). 2009. "State of Aging: 2009 State Perspectives in State Units on Aging Policies and Practices." Washington, DC: National Association of State Units on Aging.

National Governors Association. 2010. "State Roles in Delivery System Reform." Washington, DC: National Governors Association. http://www.nga.org/Files/pdf/1007deliverysystemreform.pdf.

National PACE Association. 2010. "PACE in the States." Alexandria, VA: National PACE Association.

Naylor, Mary D. 2006. "Transitional Care: A Critical Dimension of the Home Health-care Quality Agenda." *Journal for Healthcare Quality* 28(1): 48–54.

Ng, Terence, Charlene Harrington, and Molly O'Malley Watts. 2009. "Medicaid Home and Community-Based Service Programs: Data Update." Washington, DC: Kaiser Family Foundation. http://www.kff.org/medicaid/upload/7720-03.pdf.

Ng, Terence, Charlene Harrington, and Martin Kitchener. 2010. "Medicare and Medicaid in Long-Term Care." *Health Affairs* 29(1): 22–28.

North Carolina Institute of Medicine. 2007. "Task Force on the North Carolina Nursing Workforce Report: Update 2007." Raleigh, NC: North Carolina Institute of Medicine.

O'Shaughnessy, Carol V. 2009. "The Role of Ombudsmen in Assuring Quality for Residents of Long-Term Care Facilities: Straining to Make Ends Meet." Washington, DC: National Health Policy Forum.

Office the Inspector General (OIG). 1999. Long-Term Care Ombudsman Program: Overall Capacity. OIE-02-98-00351. Washington, DC: Office of the Inspector General, U.S. Department of Health and Human Services. http://www.oig.hhs.gov/oei/reports/oei-02-98-00351.pdf.

———. 2008. "Deficiency History and Recertification of Medicare Home Health Agencies." OEI-09-06-00040. Washington, DC: Office of the Inspector General, U.S. Department of Health and Human Services. http://oig.hhs.gov/oei/reports/oei-09-06-00040.pdf.

Paraprofessional Healthcare Institute (PHI). 2009. "Who Are Direct Care Workers? Fact 3." New York: Paraprofessional Healthcare Institute.

———. 2010. "Who Are the Direct Care Workers? February 2010 Update." New York: Paraprofessional Healthcare Institute. http://www.directcareclearinghouse.org/download/NCDCW%20Fact%20Sheet-1.pdf.

Picone, Gabriel, R. Mark Wilson, and Shin-Yi Chou. 2003. "Analysis of Hospital Length of Stay and Discharge Destination Using Hazard Functions with Unmeasured Heterogeneity." *Health Economics* 12(12): 1021–34.

Pinquart, Martin, and Silvia Sorensen. 2003. "Differences between Caregivers and Noncaregivers in Psychological Health and Physical Health: A Meta-Analysis." *Psychology and Aging* 18:250–67.

Population Reference Bureau. 2009. "World Population Data Sheet." Washington, DC: Population Reference Bureau. http://www.prb.org/pdf09/09wpds_eng.pdf.

Pynoos, Jon, Penny Hollander Feldman, and Joann Ahrens, eds. 2004. *Linking Housing and Services for Older Adults: Obstacles, Options, and Opportunities.* New York: Haworth Press.

Rabig, Judith, William Thomas, Rosalie A. Kane, Lois J. Cutler, and Steve McAlilly. 2006. "Radical Redesign of Nursing Homes: Applying the Green House Concept in Tupelo, Mississippi." *The Gerontologist* 46(4): 533–39.

Redfoot, Donald L., and Ari N. Houser. 2005. "'We Shall Travel On': Quality of Care, Economic Development, and the International Migration of Long-Term Care Workers." Paper No. 2005-14. Washington, DC: AARP Public Policy Institute.

Redfoot, Donald L., and Sheel M. Pandya. 2002. "Before the Boom: Trends in Long-Term Supportive Services for Older Americans with Disabilities." Washington, DC: AARP Public Policy Institute.

Reinhard, Susan C. 2010. "Diversion, Transition Programs Target Nursing Homes' Status Quo." *Health Affairs* 29(1): 44–48.

Reinhard, Susan C., Heather Young, Rosalie A. Kane, and Winifred V. Quinn. 2003. "Nurse Delegation of Medication Administration of Elders." Washington, DC: Center for Excellence in Assisted Living. http://www.theceal.org/downloads/CEAL_1177377300.pdf.

Reuben, David B. 2007. "The 21st Century American Geriatrics Society: Destinations and Highways to Get There." *Journal of the American Geriatrics Society* 55(3): 325–26.

Rollow, William, Terry R. Lied, Paul McGann, James Poyer, Lawrence LaVoie, Robert T. Kambic, Dale W. Bratzler, Allen Ma, Edwin D. Huff, and Lawrence D. Ramunno. 2006. "Assessment of the Medicare Quality Improvement Organization Program." *Annals of Internal Medicine* 145(5): 342–53.

Rosenfield, Peri, Mia Kobayashi, Patricia Barber, and Mathy Mezey. 2004. "Utilization of Nurse Practitioners in Long-Term Care: Findings and Implications of a National Survey." *Journal of the American Medical Director Association* 5(1): 9–15.

SCAN Foundation and Avalere Health. 2010. "Long-Term Care Policy Simulator." Long Beach, CA: SCAN Foundation. http://www.ltcpolicysimulator.org.

Schlenker, Robert E., David F. Hittle, and Angela G. Arnold. 1995. "Home Health Agency Quality: Medicare Certification Findings Compared to Patient Outcomes." *Home Health Care Services Quarterly* 15(4): 97–115.

Schmitt, Eva M., Laura P. Sands, Sara Weiss, Glenna Dowling, and Kenneth Lovinsky. 2010. "Adult Day Health Center Participation and Health-Related Quality of Life." *The Gerontologist* 50(4): 531–40.

Schnelle, John F., Joseph G. Ouslander, and Patrice A. Cruise. 1997. "Policy without Technology: A Barrier to Improving Nursing Home Care." *The Gerontologist* 37(4): 527–32.

Schoeni, Robert F., Vicki A. Freedman, and Robert B. Wallace. 2001. "Persistent, Consistent, Widespread, and Robust? Another Look at Recent Trends in Old-Age Disability." *Journal of Gerontology: Social Sciences* 56B(4): S206–18.

Schore, Jennifer, Leslie Foster, and Barbara Phillips. 2007. "Consumer Enrollment and Experiences in the Cash and Counseling Program." *Health Services Research* 42(1): 446–66.

Schulz, Richard, and Paula R. Sherwood. 2008. "Physical and Mental Health Effects of Family Caregiving." *American Journal of Nursing* 108(Supplement 9): 12–26.

Shih, Anthony, Diane M. Dewar, and Thomas Hartman. 2007. "Medicare's Quality Improvement Organization Program Value in Nursing Homes." *Health Care Financing Review* 28(3): 109–116.

Shortell, Stephen M., and William A. Peck. 2006. "Enhancing the Potential of Quality Improvement Organizations to Improve Quality of Care." *Annals of Internal Medicine* 145(5): 388–89.

Shugarman, Lisa R. 2010. "Health Care Reform and Long-Term Care: The Whole Is Greater than the Sum of the Parts." *Public Policy and Aging Report* 20(2): 3–7.

Shugarman, Lisa R., and Julie A. Brown. 2006. "Nursing Home Selection: How Do Consumers Choose? Volume I: Findings from Focus Groups of Consumers and Information Intermediaries." Washington, DC: Office of Disability, Aging and Long-Term Care Policy, Office of the Assistant Secretary for Planning and Evaluation, U.S. Department of Health and Human Services. http://aspe.hhs.gov/daltcp/reports/2006/chooseI.pdf.

Shugarman, Lisa R., and Rena H. Garland. 2006. "Nursing Home Selection: How Do Consumers Choose?" Washington, DC: U.S. Department of Health and Human Services. http://aspe.hhs.gov/daltcp/reports/2006/chooseIIes.htm.

Singh, Douglas A., and Robert C. Schwab. 2000. "Predicting Turnover and Retention in Nursing Home Administrators." *The Gerontologist* 40:310–19.

Smith, David Barton, Zhanlian Feng, Mary L. Fennel, Jacqueline S. Zinn, and Vincent Mor. 2007. "Separate and Unequal: Racial Segregation and Disparities in Quality across U.S. Nursing Homes." *Health Affairs* 26(5): 1448–58.

Smith, Gary, and Beth Jackson. 2004. "Summary of Results: National Quality Inventory Survey of HCBS Waiver Programs." Tualatin, OR, and Cambridge, MA: Human Services Research Institute and the MEDSTAT Group, Inc.

Smith, Karen E. 2000. "The Status of the Retired Population, Now and in the Future." In *Social Security and the Family: Addressing Unmet Needs in an Underfunded System,* edited by Melissa M. Favreault, Frank J. Sammartino, and C. Eugene Steuerle (47–88). Washington, DC: Urban Institute Press.

Smith, Kristin, and Reagan Baughman. 2007. "Caring for America's Aging Population: A Profile of the Direct-Care Workforce." *Monthly Labor Review* 130(9): 20–25.

Smith, June, and Lynda Crawford. 2003. "Report of Findings from the Practice and Professional Issues Survey, Spring 2002." Chicago: National Council of State Boards of Nursing.

Soldo, Beth J., Olivia S. Mitchell, Rania Tfaily, and John F. McCabe. 2006. "Cross-Cohort Difference in Health on the Verge of Retirement." Working Paper 12762. Cambridge, MA: National Bureau of Economic Research.

Spector, William D., M. Rhona Limcangco, and Dana B. Mukamel. 2006. "Identifying Culture Change in Nursing Homes." New York: The Commonwealth Fund.

Spillman, Brenda C., and Kristen J. Black. 2005. "Staying the Course: Trends in Family Caregiving." Washington, DC: AARP.

Stevenson, David G. 2006. "Is a Public Reporting Approach Appropriate for Nursing Home Care?" *Journal of Health Politics, Policy, and Law* 31(4): 773–810.

———. 2008. "Planning for the Future: Long-Term Care and the 2008 Election." *New England Journal of Medicine* 358(19): 1985–7.

Stevenson, David G., and David C. Grabowski. 2010. "Sizing Up the Market for Assisted Living." *Health Affairs* 29(1): 35–43.

Stevenson, David G., and David M. Studdert. 2003. "The Rise of Nursing Home Litigation: Findings from a National Survey of Attorneys." *Health Affairs* 22(2): 219–29.

Stevenson, David G., Marc A. Cohen, Eileen J. Tell, and Brian Burwell. 2010. "The Complementarity of Public and Private Long-Term Care Coverage." *Health Affairs* 29(1): 96–101.

Stone, Robyn I. 2006a. "Emerging Issues in Long-Term Care." In *Handbook of Aging and the Social Sciences,* 6th ed., edited by Robert H. Binstock and Linda K. George (397–418). Amsterdam: Academic Press.

———. 2006b. "Common or Uncommon Agendas: Consumer Direction in the Aging and Disability Movements." In *Consumer Voice and Choice in Long-Term Care,* edited by S. R. Kunkel and V. Wellin. Springer Publishing Company.

Stone, Robyn I., and Joshua M. Wiener. 2001. "Who Will Care for Us? Addressing the Long-Term Care Workforce Crisis." Washington, DC: Urban Institute and the American Association of Homes and Services for the Aging.

Stone, Robyn I., and Susan C. Reinhard. 2007. "The Place of Assisted Living in Long-Term Care and Related Services Systems." *The Gerontologist* Special Issue 3: 23–32.

Stone, Robyn I., and Steven Dawson. 2008. "The Origins of Better Jobs, Better Care." *The Gerontologist* 48(Special Issue 1): 5–13.

Stone, Robyn I., and Mary F. Harahan. 2010. "Improving the Long-Term Care Workforce Serving Older Adults." *Health Affairs* 29(1): 109–15.

Stone, Robyn I., Mary Harahan, and Alisha Sanders. 2008. "Expanding Affordable Housing with Services for Older Adults: Challenges and Potential." In *The Assisted Living Residence: A Vision for the Future,* edited by Stephen M. Golant and Joan Hyde (329–50). Baltimore, MD: Johns Hopkins University Press.

Stone, Robyn I., Natasha Bryant, and Linda Barbarotta. 2009. "Supporting Culture Change: Working toward Smarter State Nursing Home Regulation." New York: The Commonwealth Fund. http://www.commonwealthfund.org/Content/Publications/Issue-Briefs/2009/Oct/Supporting-Culture-Change.aspx.

Stone, Robyn I., Susan C. Reinhard, Barbara Bowers, David Zimmerman, Charles D. Phillips, Catherine Hawes, Jean A. Fielding, and Nora Jacobson. 2002. "Evaluation of the Wellspring Model for Improving Nursing Home Quality." New York, NY: The Commonwealth Fund.

Thomas, William H. 1994. *The Eden Alternative: Nature, Hope and Nursing Homes.* Sherburne, NY: Eden Alternative Foundation.

Tilly, Jane, and Joshua M. Wiener. 2001. "Consumer Directed Home and Community-Based Services: Policy Issues." Washington, DC: The Urban Institute. http://www.urban.org/url.cfm?ID=310065.

Tumlinson, Anne, and Christine Aguiar. 2008. "Opportunities for Comprehensive Acute and Long-Term Care Reform." Washington, DC: Avalere Health.

Tumlinson, Anne, Christine Aguiar, and Molly O'Malley Watts. 2009. "Closing the Long-Term Care Funding Gap: The Challenge of Private Long-Term Care Insurance." Report 7829. Menlo Park, CA: Kaiser Family Foundation.

Tumlinson, Anne, Weiwen Ng, and Eric Hammelman. 2010. "The Circular Relationship between Enrollment and Premiums: Effects on the CLASS Program Act." *Public Policy and Aging Report* 20(2): 28–30.

University of Michigan. 2009. "How Older Americans Are Faring in the Recession." *University of Michigan Retirement Research Center Quarterly Newsletter* 10(4): 4. http://www.mrrc.isr.umich.edu/publications/newsletters/pdf/1009.pdf.

U.S. Census Bureau. 2003. "Labor Force, Employment, and Earnings." Washington, DC: U.S. Census Bureau. http://www.census.gov/prod/2004pubs/03statab/labor.pdf.

U.S. Department of Health and Human Services. 2003. "The Future Supply of Long-Term Care Workers in Relation to the Aging Baby Boom Generation: A Report to Congress." Washington, DC: U.S. Department of Health and Human Services. http://aspe.hhs.gov/daltcp/reports.ltcwork.pdf.

U.S. Department of Labor, Bureau of Labor Statistics. 2006. *Occupational Outlook Handbook,* 2006–2007 ed. Washington, DC: U.S. Department of Labor, Bureau of Labor Statistics. http://www.bls.gov/oco/home.htm.

———. 2010. "Career Guide to Industries, 2010–2011 Edition." Washington, DC: U.S. Department of Labor. http://www.bls.gov/oco/cg/cgs035.htm.

U.S. Department of Veterans Affairs. 2010. "The Geriatrics and Extended Care Program." Washington, DC: Department of Veterans Affairs. http://www1.va.gov/geriatrics/.

U.S. General Accounting Office (GAO). 2001. "Nursing Workforce Recruitment and Retention of Nurses and Nursing Assistants Is a Growing Concern." Testimony of William J. Scanlon. http://www.gao.gov/new.items/d01750t.pdf.

———. 2002. "Medicare Home Health Agencies: Weaknesses in Federal and State Oversight Make Potential Quality Issues." GAO-02-382. Washington, DC: U.S. General Accounting Office. http://www.gao.gov/new.items/d02382.pdf.

U.S. Government Accountability Office (GAO). 2003. "Nursing Home Quality: Prevalence of Serious Problems, while Declining, Reinforces Importance of Enhanced Oversight." GAO-03-561. Washington, DC: U.S. Government Accountability Office.

———. 2005. "Despite Increased Oversight, Challenges Remain in Ensuring High-Quality Care and Resident Safety." GAO-06-117. Washington, DC: U.S. Government Accountability Office.

———. 2007a. "Nursing Homes: Efforts to Strengthen Federal Enforcement Have Not Deterred Some Homes from Repeatedly Harming Residents." GAO-07-241. Washington, DC: U.S. Government Accountability Office.

———. 2007b. "Nursing Home Reform: Continued Attention Is Needed to Improve Quality of Care in Small but Significant Share of Homes." GAO-07-794T. Washington, DC: U.S. Government Accountability Office.

———. 2009. "Nursing Homes: CMS's Special Focus Facility Methodology Should Better Target the Most Poorly Performing Homes, which Tended to Be Chain Affiliated and For-Profit." GAO-09-689. Washington, DC: U.S. Government Accountability Office.

U.S. Senate Special Committee on Aging. 1974. "Nursing Home Care in the United States: Failure in Public Policy." Washington, DC: Government Printing Office.

Van Houten, Courtney H., and Edward C. Norton. 2008. "Informal Care and Medicare Expenditures: Testing for Heterogeneous Treatment Effects." *Journal of Health Economics* 27:134–56.

Vincent, Grayson K., and Victoria A. Velkoff. 2010. "The Next Four Decades: The Older Population in the United States: 2010 to 2050." Current Population Reports P25-1138. Washington, DC: U.S. Census Bureau.

Vladeck, Bruce C. 1982. "Understanding Long-Term Care." *New England Journal of Medicine* 307:889–90.

Walsh, Kieran. 2001. "Regulating U.S. Nursing Homes: Are We Learning from Experience?" *Health Affairs* 20(6): 128.

Weiner, Audrey S., and Judah L. Ronch, eds. 2003. *Culture Change in Long-Term Care.* New York, NY: Haworth Social Work Practice Press.

Weissert, William G., Melissa Musliner, Timothy Lesnick, and Kathleen A. Foley. 1997. "Cost Savings from Home and Community-Based Services: Arizona's Capitated Medicaid Long-Term Care Program." *Journal of Health Policy Politics and Law* 22(6): 1329–57.

Wenzlow, Audra T., and Debra J. Lipson. 2009. "Transitioning Medicaid Enrollees from Institutions to the Community: Number of People Eligible and Number of Transitions Targeted under MFP." *The National Evaluation of the Money Follows the Person Demonstration Grant Program: Reports from the Field* 1. Cambridge, MA: Mathematica Policy Research.

Werner, Rachel M., and R. Tamara Konetzka. 2010. "Advancing Nursing Home Quality through Quality Improvement Itself." *Health Affairs* 29(1): 81–86.

Wiener, Joshua M. 2009. "Long-Term Care: Options in an Era of Health Reform." Washington, DC: RTI International.

———. 2010. "What Does Health Reform Mean for Long-Term Care?" *Public Policy and Aging Report* 20(2): 8–15.

Wiener, Joshua M., Wayne L. Anderson, and Barbara Gage. 2009. "Making the System Work for Home Care Quality." *Journal of Healthcare Quality* 31(2): 18–23.

Wiener, Joshua M., Marc P. Freiman, and David Brown. 2007. "Nursing Home Care Quality: Twenty Years after the Omnibus Budget Reconciliation Act of 1987." Washington, DC: RTI International.

Wiener, Joshua M., Marie R. Squillace, Wayne L. Anderson, and Galina Khatutsky. 2009. "Why Do They Stay? Job Tenure among Certified Nursing Assistants in Nursing Homes." *The Gerontologist* 49(2): 198–210.

Wiener, Joshua M., Jane Tilly, and Susan M. Goldenson. 2000. "Federal and State Initiatives to Jump Start the Market for Private Long-Term Care Insurance." *The Elder Law Journal* 8(1): 57–102.

Williams, Judith, Barbara Lyons, and Diane Rowland. 1997. "Unmet Long-Term Care Needs of Elderly People in the Community: A Review of the Literature." *Home Health Care Services Quarterly* 16:93–119.

Wilson, Keren Brown. 2007. "Historical Evolution of Assisted Living in the United States, 1979 to the Present." *The Gerontologist* 47(Spec. 3): 8–22.

Wolf, Douglas A. 2001. "Population Change: Friend or Foe of the Chronic Care System?" *Health Affairs* 20(6): 28–42.

Wolff, Jennifer L., and Judith D. Kasper. 2006. "Caregivers of Frail Elders: Updating a National Profile." *The Gerontologist* 3:344–56.

Wu, Ning, Susan C. Miller, Kate Lapane, and Vincent Mor. 2005. "The Quality of the Quality Indicator of Pain Derived from the Minimum Data Set." *Health Services Research* 40(4): 1197–1216.

Wunderlich, Gooloo S., and Peter O. Kohler, eds. 2001. *Improving the Quality of Long-Term Care.* Washington, DC: National Academy of Sciences, Institute of Medicine.

Zimmerman, Sheryl L., Philip D. Sloane, and Susan K. Fletcher. 2008. "The Measurement and Importance of Quality: A Collaborative Effort for Tomorrow's Assisted Living." In *The Assisted Living Residence: A Vision for the Future,* edited by Stephen M. Golant and Joan Hyde (119–42). Baltimore, MD: Johns Hopkins University Press.

About the Author

Robyn Stone is a noted researcher and internationally recognized authority on long-term care and aging policy. During her 35-year career, she has held high-profile positions in the public and private sectors and has published widely on long-term care policy and quality, chronic care for the disabled, aging services workforce development, and family caregiving. Since 1999, she has served as the senior vice president for research at LeadingAge (formerly the American Association of Homes and Services for the Aging) and was the founder of the LeadingAge Center for Applied Research in Washington, D.C. She has held senior research and policy positions in the U.S. government, serving in the U.S. Department of Health and Human Services as deputy assistant secretary for disability, aging, and long-term care policy from 1993 through 1996 and as assistant secretary for aging in 1997. Dr. Stone is a distinguished national and international speaker and serves on numerous provider and nonprofit boards that focus on aging services issues.

Index